Daily Menière's Journal

The spark of HOPE
can never be extinguished.

Julieann Wallace

Lilly Pilly
PUBLISHING

3 Month Daily Meniere's Journal
Created by Julieann Wallace ©2021
Cover design by Julieann Wallace
Main cover image 123rf ID: 161166230
Published in Australia 2021 by Lilly Pilly Publishing
lillypillypublishing@outlook.com

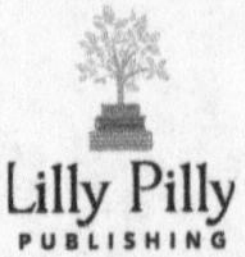

ISBN: 978-0-6451581-0-6 (print book)

About Julieann Wallace - Julieann is a bestselling, multi-published author, artist, and teacher, who is inspired by the gift of imagination and the power of words. She writes picture books under her own name, and novels under the name of Amelia Grace, where she donates money from sales to help find a cure for Meniere's disease. Julieann is a self-confessed tea ninja, Cadbury chocoholic, has a passion for music and art, and tries not to scare her cat, Claude Monet, with her terrible cello playing.

In 2018, Julieann released a novel with a main character with Meniere's disease. *The Colour of Broken* has been a global success, hitting #1 on Amazon in its category. In 2021, *The Colour of Broken* was long-listed to be made into a movie or TV series with Screen QLD. In 2021, the sequel was released, 'All the Colours Above'. Julieann has also written two Meniere's picture books Vanilla Swirl, for mothers with Meniere's disease, and Blueberry Swirl, for fathers with Meniere's disease. 100% of profits from all these books are donated to Meniere's research at the *University of Sydney's Brain and Mind Institute.*

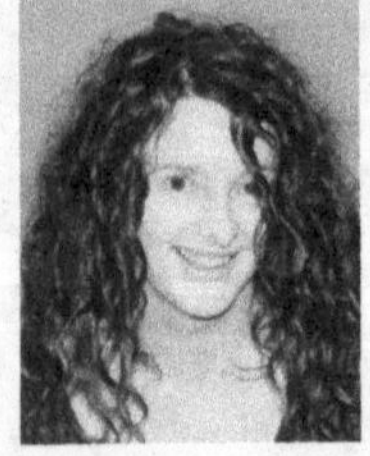

Stay up-to-date with Julieann:
Website: *www.julieannwallaceauthor.com*
Facebook: *www.facebook.com/julieannwallace.author*
Instagram: @julieann_wallace_
Instagram: @myshadow_menieres
Follow Julieann's blog, **My Shadow, Meniere's:**
www.myshadowmenieres.wordpress.com

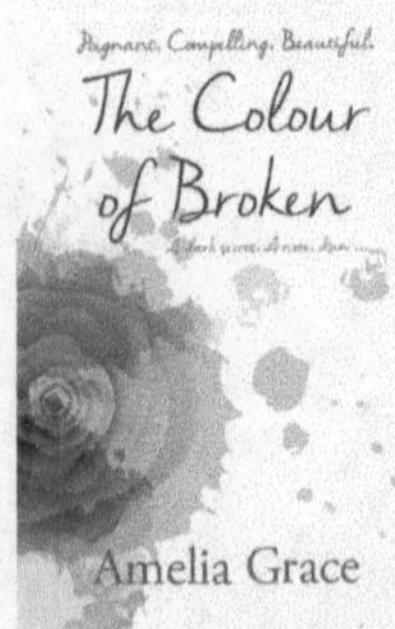

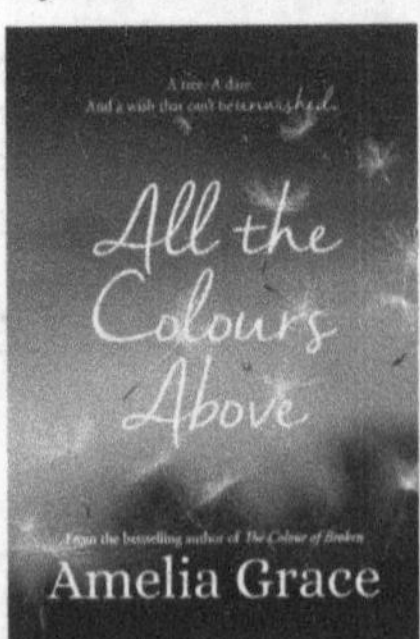

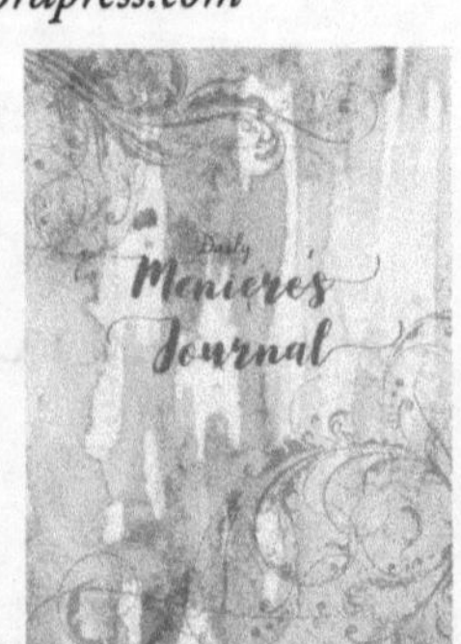

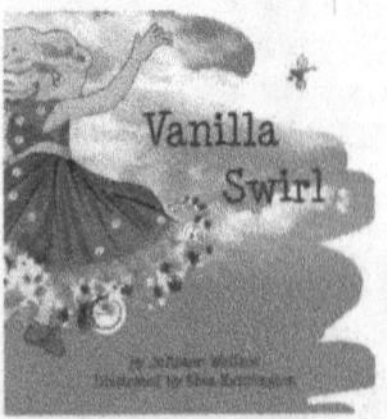

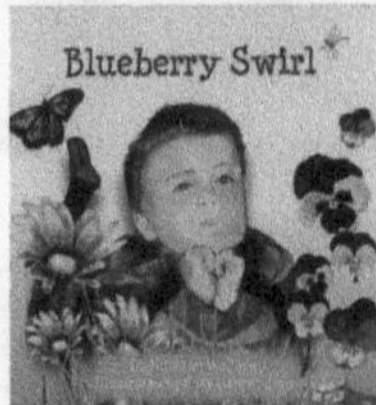

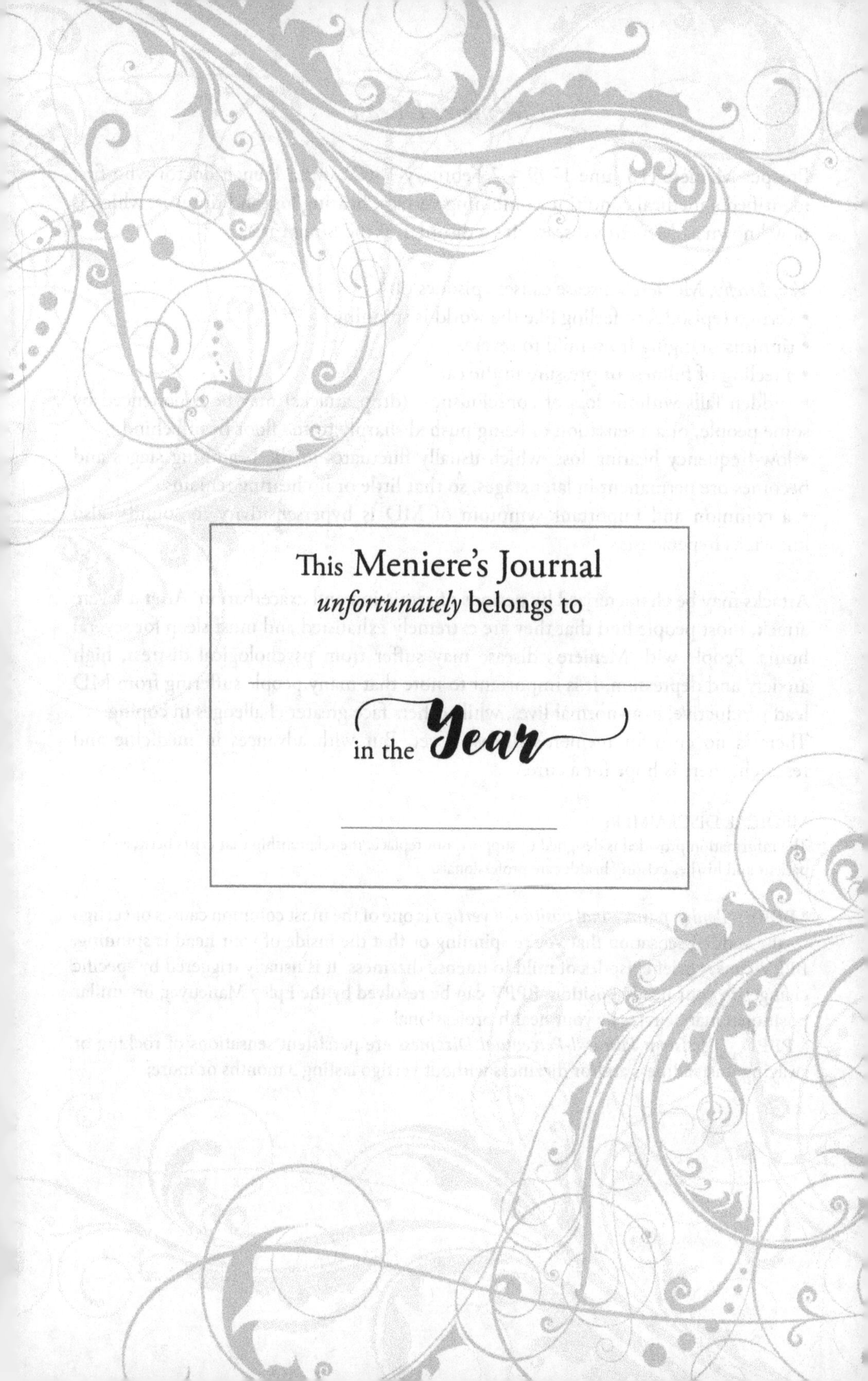

This Meniere's Journal *unfortunately* belongs to

____

in the Year

____

Meniere's Disease

Prosper Menière (18 June 1799 – 7 February 1862) was a French doctor who first identified a medical condition combining vertigo, hearing loss and tinnitus, which is now known as Menière's disease. It's a disorder of the inner ear.

Very briefly, Meniere's disease causes episodes of:
• vertigo (episodes of feeling like the world is spinning)
• tinnitus - ranging from mild to severe.
• a feeling of fullness or pressure in the ear.
• sudden falls without loss of consciousness (drop attacks) may be experienced by some people, or a a sensation of being pushed sharply to the floor from behind.
• low-frequency hearing loss, which usually fluctuates in the beginning stages and becomes ore permanent in later stages, so that little or no hearing remains.
• a common and important symptom of MD is hypersensitivity to sounds, also known as hyperacusis.

Attacks may be characterized by periods of remission and exacerbation. After a severe attack, most people find that they are extremely exhausted and must sleep for several hours. People with Meniere's disease may suffer from psychological distress, high anxiety and depression. It is important to note that many people suffering from MD lead productive, near-normal lives, while others face greater challenges in coping. There is no cure for meniere's disease - yet. But with advances in medicine and research, there is hope for a cure.

MEDICAL DISCLAIMER:
The information provided is designed to support, not replace, the relationship that exists between a patient and his/her existing health care professionals.

* **BPPV** - *Benign paroxysmal positional vertigo* is one of the most common causes of vertigo — the sudden sensation that you're spinning or that the inside of your head is spinning. BPPV causes brief episodes of mild to intense dizziness. It is usually triggered by specific changes in your head's position. BPPV can be resolved by the Epley Maneuver, or similar positional manoeuvres by your health professional.
* **PPPD** - *Persistent Postural-Perceptual Dizziness* are persistent sensations of rocking or swaying unsteadiness and/or dizziness without vertigo lasting 3 months or more;

About the

Daily Meniere's Journal

My shadow, Meniere's, has been with me for 26 years at the time of this journal publication. A very difficult first 10 years, where I would be debilitated for 4 hours or more at a time with horrendous violent vertigo at least 40 times a year. Meniere's an absolute life changer. I developed a chronic fear of vertigo attacks, and PTSD, and so stopped shopping, socialising, driving, and teaching. Everyday I kept a diary of what I ate or drank, where I had been and what I had done, to see if I could find the trigger for my attacks.

It is my hope that this journal can help you. By keeping a track of your daily living with Meniere's, you may find a pattern that will help you with your battle against it. As you are using the journal, highlight symptoms you have on that day, add notes about what you are experiencing, or any new symptoms, plus vertigo length and severity. Please be aware that I have added BPPV* (Benign Paroxysmal Positional Vertigo - a problem with the crystals in the inner ear - symptoms are brief periods of vertigo, that is, of a spinning sensation upon changes in the position of the head, lasting less than a minute). BPPV is **NOT** a symptom of Meniere's. You can have Meniere's and BPPV at the same time. BPPV has a technique called the *Epley Manoeuvre* that can stop those episodes.

Because this is your journal, you can add your own stamp and style. Glue in prayers, inspirational verses or images that speak to you in some way. Be creative, be arty. I have added pages of light text at the end of each month, where you can draw or paint artwork over the top, or glue notes you have written, or letters to yourself etc. Being a Secondary Art Teacher, I know the value of art as a tool for healing and restoration, when words are simply not enough.

Three Things I am Thankful for Today - When I was struggling in a deep and dark depression with my Meniere's in the early 2000's, I learned the value of finding things I was thankful for. *Everyday. Single. Day.* No matter how small. This act of focusing is now called 'Mindfulness', and is very powerful. As you travel daily with your Meniere's, remember, **you are a warrior. You've got this!**

It is my forever hope and prayer, that a cure is found.

Julieann xo

MONTH: January February March April May June July August September October November December

Day: Monday Tuesday Wednesday Thursday Friday Saturday Sunday

Date: ______ **Season:** Summer Autumn/Fall Winter Spring

Temperature: Low ______ High ______

Barometer: 9am ______ 9pm ______ **Humidity** ______

Sunny	Cloudy	Rain	Showers	Windy
Snow	Storm	Humid	Dry	

Food & Fluid Intake (be mindful of salt):

Breakfast			
Lunch			
Dinner			
Fluid Intake	Water - ______		
Snacks			

Symptoms:

Tinnitus	Vertigo	Drop Attack	Nausea
Anxiety	Brain Fog	Hearing Loss	Hyperacusis
Fatigue	Balance	Co-ordination	Stress
Headache	Migraine	Nystagmus	Disequilibrium
Ear Fullness/ Pressure/Pain	Vision Difficulties	Physical Impairment	Vestibular Migraine
Vomiting	Depression	BPPV*	Diarrhea
PPPD*	Jaw Click/Pain	Neck Pain	Motion Sensitivity
Sweating	Speech Difficulty	Monthly Cycle	

What time did your symptoms start? ______________________

Tinnitus: L R How many noises? ________ Loudness Scale: 1 2 3 4 5

Possible Meniere's Symptom Triggers Today:

Physical: ____

____

____

__________________________ Pollen, Mold, Dust, Trees, Grass, Ragweed

Visual: ____

____

____

Emotional: ____

____

____

What Helped Me?

Medication/s & Time Taken		Other	
		Prayer	Rest
		Meditation	Friend/s
		Self-care	Family
		Exercise	Pet/s
		Mindfulness	Vestibular Rehab
		Gratitude	Hearing Device

Duration of Vertigo _______ minutes _______ hours_______ days

Severity of Vertigo 1 2 3 4 5 - I HATE you, vertigo!

New Symptoms? ______________________________________

____

What I Accomplished Today - Something to Celebrate! ♡

____

____

____

Three Things I am Thankful for Today:

1.
2.
3.

MONTH: January February March April May June July August September October November December

Day: Monday Tuesday Wednesday Thursday Friday Saturday Sunday

Date: ______ **Season:** Summer Autumn/Fall Winter Spring

Temperature: Low ______ High ______

Barometer: 9am________ 9pm________ **Humidity** __________

Sunny	Cloudy	Rain	Showers	Windy
Snow	Storm	Humid	Dry	

Food & Fluid Intake (be mindful of salt):

Breakfast			
Lunch			
Dinner			
Fluid Intake	Water -		
Snacks			

Symptoms:

Tinnitus	Vertigo	Drop Attack	Nausea
Anxiety	Brain Fog	Hearing Loss	Hyperacusis
Fatigue	Balance	Co-ordination	Stress
Headache	Migraine	Nystagmus	Disequilibrium
Ear Fullness/ Pressure/Pain	Vision Difficulties	Physical Impairment	Vestibular Migraine
Vomiting	Depression	BPPV*	Diarrhea
PPPD*	Jaw Click/Pain	Neck Pain	Motion Sensitivity
Sweating	Speech Difficulty	Monthly Cycle	

What time did your symptoms start? ____________________

Tinnitus: L R How many noises? ______ Loudness Scale: 1 2 3 4 5

Possible Meniere's Symptom Triggers Today:

Physical: ____________________

____

____

____________________ Pollen, Mold, Dust, Trees, Grass, Ragweed

Visual: ____________________

____

____

Emotional: ____________________

____

____

What Helped Me?

Medication/s & Time Taken		Other	
		Prayer	Rest
		Meditation	Friend/s
		Self-care	Family
		Exercise	Pet/s
		Mindfulness	Vestibular Rehab
		Gratitude	Hearing Device

Duration of Vertigo ______ minutes ______ hours ______ days

Severity of Vertigo 1 2 3 4 5 - I HATE you, vertigo!

New Symptoms? ____________________

____

What I Accomplished Today – Something to Celebrate! ♡

____

____

____

Three Things I am Thankful for Today:

1.
2.
3.

MONTH: January February March April May June July August September October November December

Day: Monday Tuesday Wednesday Thursday Friday Saturday Sunday
Date: ______ **Season:** Summer Autumn/Fall Winter Spring
Temperature: Low _______ High _______
Barometer: 9am__________ 9pm__________ **Humidity** __________

Sunny	Cloudy	Rain	Showers	Windy
Snow	Storm	Humid	Dry	

Food & Fluid Intake (be mindful of salt):

Breakfast			
Lunch			
Dinner			
Fluid Intake	Water - ______		
Snacks			

Symptoms:

Tinnitus	Vertigo	Drop Attack	Nausea
Anxiety	Brain Fog	Hearing Loss	Hyperacusis
Fatigue	Balance	Co-ordination	Stress
Headache	Migraine	Nystagmus	Disequilibrium
Ear Fullness/ Pressure/Pain	Vision Difficulties	Physical Impairment	Vestibular Migraine
Vomiting	Depression	BPPV*	Diarrhea
PPPD*	Jaw Click/Pain	Neck Pain	Motion Sensitivity
Sweating	Speech Difficulty	Monthly Cycle	

What time did your symptoms start? ____________________

Tinnitus: L R How many noises? ______ Loudness Scale: 1 2 3 4 5

Possible Meniere's Symptom Triggers Today:

Physical: ____________________

____

____

____________________ Pollen, Mold, Dust, Trees, Grass, Ragweed

Visual: ____________________

____

____

Emotional: ____________________

____

____

What Helped Me?

Medication/s & Time Taken		Other	
		Prayer	Rest
		Meditation	Friend/s
		Self-care	Family
		Exercise	Pet/s
		Mindfulness	Vestibular Rehab
		Gratitude	Hearing Device

Duration of Vertigo ______ minutes ______ hours ______ days

Severity of Vertigo 1 2 3 4 5 - I HATE you, vertigo!

New Symptoms? ____________________

____

What I Accomplished Today – Something to Celebrate! ♡

____

____

____

Three Things I am Thankful for Today:

1.
2.
3.

MONTH: January February March April May June July August September October November December

Day: Monday Tuesday Wednesday Thursday Friday Saturday Sunday
Date: ______ **Season:** Summer Autumn/Fall Winter Spring
Temperature: Low ______ High ______
Barometer: 9am ______ 9pm ______ **Humidity** ______

Sunny	Cloudy	Rain	Showers	Windy
Snow	Storm	Humid	Dry	

Food & Fluid Intake (be mindful of salt):

Breakfast			
Lunch			
Dinner			
Fluid Intake	Water - ______		
Snacks			

Symptoms:

Tinnitus	Vertigo	Drop Attack	Nausea
Anxiety	Brain Fog	Hearing Loss	Hyperacusis
Fatigue	Balance	Co-ordination	Stress
Headache	Migraine	Nystagmus	Disequilibrium
Ear Fullness/ Pressure/Pain	Vision Difficulties	Physical Impairment	Vestibular Migraine
Vomiting	Depression	BPPV*	Diarrhea
PPPD*	Jaw Click/Pain	Neck Pain	Motion Sensitivity
Sweating	Speech Difficulty	Monthly Cycle	

What time did your symptoms start? ____________________

Tinnitus: L R How many noises? _______ Loudness Scale: 1 2 3 4 5

Possible Meniere's Symptom Triggers Today:

Physical: ____________________

____

____

____________________ Pollen, Mold, Dust, Trees, Grass, Ragweed

Visual: ____________________

____

____

Emotional: ____________________

____

____

What Helped Me?

Medication/s & Time Taken		Other	
		Prayer	Rest
		Meditation	Friend/s
		Self-care	Family
		Exercise	Pet/s
		Mindfulness	Vestibular Rehab
		Gratitude	Hearing Device

Duration of Vertigo ______ minutes ______ hours______ days

Severity of Vertigo 1 2 3 4 5 - I HATE you, vertigo!

New Symptoms? ____________________

____

What I Accomplished Today - Something to Celebrate! ♡

____

____

____

Three Things I am Thankful for Today:

1.
2.
3.

MONTH: January February March April May June July August September October November December

Day: Monday Tuesday Wednesday Thursday Friday Saturday Sunday

Date: ______ **Season:** Summer Autumn/Fall Winter Spring

Temperature: Low _______ High _______

Barometer: 9am_________ 9pm________ **Humidity** ___________

Sunny	Cloudy	Rain	Showers	Windy
Snow	Storm	Humid	Dry	

Food & Fluid Intake (be mindful of salt):

Breakfast			
Lunch			
Dinner			
Fluid Intake	Water -		
Snacks			

Symptoms:

Tinnitus	Vertigo	Drop Attack	Nausea
Anxiety	Brain Fog	Hearing Loss	Hyperacusis
Fatigue	Balance	Co-ordination	Stress
Headache	Migraine	Nystagmus	Disequilibrium
Ear Fullness/ Pressure/Pain	Vision Difficulties	Physical Impairment	Vestibular Migraine
Vomiting	Depression	BPPV*	Diarrhea
PPPD*	Jaw Click/Pain	Neck Pain	Motion Sensitivity
Sweating	Speech Difficulty	Monthly Cycle	

What time did your symptoms start? ____________

Tinnitus: L R How many noises? ______ Loudness Scale: 1 2 3 4 5

Possible Meniere's Symptom Triggers Today:

Physical: ____________

____

____

____________ Pollen, Mold, Dust, Trees, Grass, Ragweed

Visual: ____________

____

____

Emotional: ____________

____

____

What Helped Me?

Medication/s & Time Taken		Other	
		Prayer	Rest
		Meditation	Friend/s
		Self-care	Family
		Exercise	Pet/s
		Mindfulness	Vestibular Rehab
		Gratitude	Hearing Device

Duration of Vertigo _____ minutes _____ hours_____ days

Severity of Vertigo 1 2 3 4 5 - I HATE you, vertigo!

New Symptoms? ____________

____

What I Accomplished Today – Something to Celebrate! ♡

____

____

____

Three Things I am Thankful for Today:

1.
2.
3.

MONTH: January February March April May June July August September October November December

Day: Monday Tuesday Wednesday Thursday Friday Saturday Sunday
Date: ______ **Season:** Summer Autumn/Fall Winter Spring
Temperature: Low ______ High ______
Barometer: 9am______ 9pm______ **Humidity** ______

Sunny	Cloudy	Rain	Showers	Windy
Snow	Storm	Humid	Dry	

Food & Fluid Intake (be mindful of salt):

Breakfast			
Lunch			
Dinner			
Fluid Intake	Water - ______		
Snacks			

Symptoms:

Tinnitus	Vertigo	Drop Attack	Nausea
Anxiety	Brain Fog	Hearing Loss	Hyperacusis
Fatigue	Balance	Co-ordination	Stress
Headache	Migraine	Nystagmus	Disequilibrium
Ear Fullness/ Pressure/Pain	Vision Difficulties	Physical Impairment	Vestibular Migraine
Vomiting	Depression	BPPV*	Diarrhea
PPPD*	Jaw Click/Pain	Neck Pain	Motion Sensitivity
Sweating	Speech Difficulty	Monthly Cycle	

What time did your symptoms start? ____________________

Tinnitus: L R How many noises? ______ Loudness Scale: 1 2 3 4 5

Possible Meniere's Symptom Triggers Today:

Physical: ____________________

____

____

____________________ Pollen, Mold, Dust, Trees, Grass, Ragweed

Visual: ____________________

____

____

Emotional: ____________________

____

____

What Helped Me?

Medication/s & Time Taken		Other	
		Prayer	Rest
		Meditation	Friend/s
		Self-care	Family
		Exercise	Pet/s
		Mindfulness	Vestibular Rehab
		Gratitude	Hearing Device

Duration of Vertigo ______ minutes ______ hours______ days

Severity of Vertigo 1 2 3 4 5 - I HATE you, vertigo!

New Symptoms? ____________________

____

What I Accomplished Today – Something to Celebrate! ♡

____

____

____

Three Things I am Thankful for Today:

1.
2.
3.

MONTH: January February March April May June July August September October November December

Day: Monday Tuesday Wednesday Thursday Friday Saturday Sunday
Date: ______ **Season:** Summer Autumn/Fall Winter Spring
Temperature: Low ______ High ______
Barometer: 9am______ 9pm______ **Humidity** ______

Sunny	Cloudy	Rain	Showers	Windy
Snow	Storm	Humid	Dry	

Food & Fluid Intake (be mindful of salt):

Breakfast			
Lunch			
Dinner			
Fluid Intake	Water - ______		
Snacks			

Symptoms:

Tinnitus	Vertigo	Drop Attack	Nausea
Anxiety	Brain Fog	Hearing Loss	Hyperacusis
Fatigue	Balance	Co-ordination	Stress
Headache	Migraine	Nystagmus	Disequilibrium
Ear Fullness/ Pressure/Pain	Vision Difficulties	Physical Impairment	Vestibular Migraine
Vomiting	Depression	BPPV*	Diarrhea
PPPD*	Jaw Click/Pain	Neck Pain	Motion Sensitivity
Sweating	Speech Difficulty	Monthly Cycle	

What time did your symptoms start? ____________________

Tinnitus: L R How many noises? ________ Loudness Scale: 1 2 3 4 5

Possible Meniere's Symptom Triggers Today:

Physical: ____________________

____

____

____________________ Pollen, Mold, Dust, Trees, Grass, Ragweed

Visual: ____________________

____

____

Emotional: ____________________

____

____

What Helped Me?

Medication/s & Time Taken		Other	
		Prayer	Rest
		Meditation	Friend/s
		Self-care	Family
		Exercise	Pet/s
		Mindfulness	Vestibular Rehab
		Gratitude	Hearing Device

Duration of Vertigo ______ minutes ______ hours ______ days

Severity of Vertigo 1 2 3 4 5 - I HATE you, vertigo!

New Symptoms? ____________________

____

What I Accomplished Today – Something to Celebrate! ♡

____

____

____

Three Things I am Thankful for Today:

1.
2.
3.

MONTH: January February March April May June July August September October November December

Day: Monday Tuesday Wednesday Thursday Friday Saturday Sunday

Date: ______ **Season:** Summer Autumn/Fall Winter Spring

Temperature: Low _______ High _______

Barometer: 9am________ 9pm________ **Humidity** ___________

Sunny	Cloudy	Rain	Showers	Windy
Snow	Storm	Humid	Dry	

Food & Fluid Intake (be mindful of salt):

Breakfast			
Lunch			
Dinner			
Fluid Intake	Water - ______		
Snacks			

Symptoms:

Tinnitus	Vertigo	Drop Attack	Nausea
Anxiety	Brain Fog	Hearing Loss	Hyperacusis
Fatigue	Balance	Co-ordination	Stress
Headache	Migraine	Nystagmus	Disequilibrium
Ear Fullness/ Pressure/Pain	Vision Difficulties	Physical Impairment	Vestibular Migraine
Vomiting	Depression	BPPV*	Diarrhea
PPPD*	Jaw Click/Pain	Neck Pain	Motion Sensitivity
Sweating	Speech Difficulty	Monthly Cycle	

What time did your symptoms start? ______

Tinnitus: L R How many noises? ______ Loudness Scale: 1 2 3 4 5

Possible Meniere's Symptom Triggers Today:

Physical: ______

______ Pollen, Mold, Dust, Trees, Grass, Ragweed

Visual: ______

Emotional: ______

What Helped Me?

Medication/s & Time Taken		Other	
		Prayer	Rest
		Meditation	Friend/s
		Self-care	Family
		Exercise	Pet/s
		Mindfulness	Vestibular Rehab
		Gratitude	Hearing Device

Duration of Vertigo ______ minutes ______ hours ______ days

Severity of Vertigo 1 2 3 4 5 - I HATE you, vertigo!

New Symptoms? ______

What I Accomplished Today - Something to Celebrate! ♡

______

Three Things I am Thankful for Today:

1.
2.
3.

MONTH: January February March April May June July August September October November December

Day: Monday Tuesday Wednesday Thursday Friday Saturday Sunday
Date: ______ **Season:** Summer Autumn/Fall Winter Spring
Temperature: Low ______ High ______
Barometer: 9am______ 9pm______ **Humidity** ______

Sunny	Cloudy	Rain	Showers	Windy
Snow	Storm	Humid	Dry	

Food & Fluid Intake (be mindful of salt):

Breakfast			
Lunch			
Dinner			
Fluid Intake	Water - ______		
Snacks			

Symptoms:

Tinnitus	Vertigo	Drop Attack	Nausea
Anxiety	Brain Fog	Hearing Loss	Hyperacusis
Fatigue	Balance	Co-ordination	Stress
Headache	Migraine	Nystagmus	Disequilibrium
Ear Fullness/ Pressure/Pain	Vision Difficulties	Physical Impairment	Vestibular Migraine
Vomiting	Depression	BPPV*	Diarrhea
PPPD*	Jaw Click/Pain	Neck Pain	Motion Sensitivity
Sweating	Speech Difficulty	Monthly Cycle	

What time did your symptoms start? ____________________

Tinnitus: L R How many noises? ______ Loudness Scale: 1 2 3 4 5

Possible Meniere's Symptom Triggers Today:

Physical: ____________________

____

____

____________________ Pollen, Mold, Dust, Trees, Grass, Ragweed

Visual: ____________________

____

____

Emotional: ____________________

____

____

What Helped Me?

Medication/s & Time Taken		Other	
		Prayer	Rest
		Meditation	Friend/s
		Self-care	Family
		Exercise	Pet/s
		Mindfulness	Vestibular Rehab
		Gratitude	Hearing Device

Duration of Vertigo ______ minutes ______ hours ______ days

Severity of Vertigo 1 2 3 4 5 - I HATE you, vertigo!

New Symptoms? ____________________

____

What I Accomplished Today – Something to Celebrate! ♡

____

____

____

Three Things I am Thankful for Today:

1.
2.
3.

MONTH: January February March April May June July August September October November December

Day: Monday Tuesday Wednesday Thursday Friday Saturday Sunday

Date: ______ **Season:** Summer Autumn/Fall Winter Spring

Temperature: Low _______ High _______

Barometer: 9am_________ 9pm_________ **Humidity** ___________

Sunny	Cloudy	Rain	Showers	Windy
Snow	Storm	Humid	Dry	

Food & Fluid Intake (be mindful of salt):

Breakfast			
Lunch			
Dinner			
Fluid Intake	Water - ______		
Snacks			

Symptoms:

Tinnitus	Vertigo	Drop Attack	Nausea
Anxiety	Brain Fog	Hearing Loss	Hyperacusis
Fatigue	Balance	Co-ordination	Stress
Headache	Migraine	Nystagmus	Disequilibrium
Ear Fullness/ Pressure/Pain	Vision Difficulties	Physical Impairment	Vestibular Migraine
Vomiting	Depression	BPPV*	Diarrhea
PPPD*	Jaw Click/Pain	Neck Pain	Motion Sensitivity
Sweating	Speech Difficulty	Monthly Cycle	

What time did your symptoms start? ____________________

Tinnitus: L R How many noises? ________ Loudness Scale: 1 2 3 4 5

Possible Meniere's Symptom Triggers Today:

Physical: ____________________

____

____

____________________ Pollen, Mold, Dust, Trees, Grass, Ragweed

Visual: ____________________

____

____

Emotional: ____________________

____

____

What Helped Me?

Medication/s & Time Taken		Other	
		Prayer	Rest
		Meditation	Friend/s
		Self-care	Family
		Exercise	Pet/s
		Mindfulness	Vestibular Rehab
		Gratitude	Hearing Device

Duration of Vertigo ______ minutes ______ hours______ days

Severity of Vertigo 1 2 3 4 5 - I HATE you, vertigo!

New Symptoms? ____________________

____

What I Accomplished Today – Something to Celebrate! ♡

____

____

____

Three Things I am Thankful for Today:

1.
2.
3.

MONTH: January February March April May June July August September October November December

Day: Monday Tuesday Wednesday Thursday Friday Saturday Sunday
Date: ______ **Season:** Summer Autumn/Fall Winter Spring
Temperature: Low _______ High _______
Barometer: 9am_________ 9pm________ **Humidity** ___________

Sunny	Cloudy	Rain	Showers	Windy
Snow	Storm	Humid	Dry	

Food & Fluid Intake (be mindful of salt):

Breakfast			
Lunch			
Dinner			
Fluid Intake	Water - ______		
Snacks			

Symptoms:

Tinnitus	Vertigo	Drop Attack	Nausea
Anxiety	Brain Fog	Hearing Loss	Hyperacusis
Fatigue	Balance	Co-ordination	Stress
Headache	Migraine	Nystagmus	Disequilibrium
Ear Fullness/ Pressure/Pain	Vision Difficulties	Physical Impairment	Vestibular Migraine
Vomiting	Depression	BPPV*	Diarrhea
PPPD*	Jaw Click/Pain	Neck Pain	Motion Sensitivity
Sweating	Speech Difficulty	Monthly Cycle	

What time did your symptoms start? ____________________

Tinnitus: L R How many noises? _______ Loudness Scale: 1 2 3 4 5

Possible Meniere's Symptom Triggers Today:

Physical: ____________________

____

____

____________________ Pollen, Mold, Dust, Trees, Grass, Ragweed

Visual: ____________________

____

____

Emotional: ____________________

____

____

What Helped Me?

Medication/s & Time Taken		Other	
		Prayer	Rest
		Meditation	Friend/s
		Self-care	Family
		Exercise	Pet/s
		Mindfulness	Vestibular Rehab
		Gratitude	Hearing Device

Duration of Vertigo ______ minutes ______ hours ______ days

Severity of Vertigo 1 2 3 4 5 - I HATE you, vertigo!

New Symptoms? ____________________

____

What I Accomplished Today - Something to Celebrate! ♡

____

____

____

Three Things I am Thankful for Today:

1.
2.
3.

MONTH: January February March April May June July August September October November December

Day: Monday Tuesday Wednesday Thursday Friday Saturday Sunday
Date: ______ **Season:** Summer Autumn/Fall Winter Spring
Temperature: Low ______ High ______
Barometer: 9am ______ 9pm ______ **Humidity** ______

Sunny	Cloudy	Rain	Showers	Windy
Snow	Storm	Humid	Dry	

Food & Fluid Intake (be mindful of salt):

Breakfast			
Lunch			
Dinner			
Fluid Intake	Water - ______		
Snacks			

Symptoms:

Tinnitus	Vertigo	Drop Attack	Nausea
Anxiety	Brain Fog	Hearing Loss	Hyperacusis
Fatigue	Balance	Co-ordination	Stress
Headache	Migraine	Nystagmus	Disequilibrium
Ear Fullness/ Pressure/Pain	Vision Difficulties	Physical Impairment	Vestibular Migraine
Vomiting	Depression	BPPV*	Diarrhea
PPPD*	Jaw Click/Pain	Neck Pain	Motion Sensitivity
Sweating	Speech Difficulty	Monthly Cycle	

What time did your symptoms start? ____________________

Tinnitus: L R How many noises? ______ Loudness Scale: 1 2 3 4 5

Possible Meniere's Symptom Triggers Today:

Physical: ____________________

____

____

____________________ Pollen, Mold, Dust, Trees, Grass, Ragweed

Visual: ____________________

____

____

Emotional: ____________________

____

____

What Helped Me?

Medication/s & Time Taken		Other	
		Prayer	Rest
		Meditation	Friend/s
		Self-care	Family
		Exercise	Pet/s
		Mindfulness	Vestibular Rehab
		Gratitude	Hearing Device

Duration of Vertigo ______ minutes ______ hours ______ days

Severity of Vertigo 1 2 3 4 5 - I HATE you, vertigo!

New Symptoms? ____________________

____

What I Accomplished Today – Something to Celebrate! ♡

____

____

____

Three Things I am Thankful for Today:

1.
2.
3.

MONTH: January February March April May June July August September October November December

Day: Monday Tuesday Wednesday Thursday Friday Saturday Sunday
Date: ______ **Season:** Summer Autumn/Fall Winter Spring
Temperature: Low ______ High ______
Barometer: 9am______ 9pm______ **Humidity** ______

Sunny	Cloudy	Rain	Showers	Windy
Snow	Storm	Humid	Dry	

Food & Fluid Intake (be mindful of salt):

Breakfast			
Lunch			
Dinner			
Fluid Intake	Water - ____		
Snacks			

Symptoms:

Tinnitus	Vertigo	Drop Attack	Nausea
Anxiety	Brain Fog	Hearing Loss	Hyperacusis
Fatigue	Balance	Co-ordination	Stress
Headache	Migraine	Nystagmus	Disequilibrium
Ear Fullness/ Pressure/Pain	Vision Difficulties	Physical Impairment	Vestibular Migraine
Vomiting	Depression	BPPV*	Diarrhea
PPPD*	Jaw Click/Pain	Neck Pain	Motion Sensitivity
Sweating	Speech Difficulty	Monthly Cycle	

What time did your symptoms start? ____________________

Tinnitus: L R How many noises? _______ Loudness Scale: 1 2 3 4 5

Possible Meniere's Symptom Triggers Today:

Physical: ____________________

____________________ Pollen, Mold, Dust, Trees, Grass, Ragweed

Visual: ____________________

Emotional: ____________________

What Helped Me?

Medication/s & Time Taken		Other	
		Prayer	Rest
		Meditation	Friend/s
		Self-care	Family
		Exercise	Pet/s
		Mindfulness	Vestibular Rehab
		Gratitude	Hearing Device

Duration of Vertigo ______ minutes ______ hours______ days

Severity of Vertigo 1 2 3 4 5 - I HATE you, vertigo!

New Symptoms? ____________________

What I Accomplished Today - Something to Celebrate! ♡

Three Things I am Thankful for Today:

1.
2.
3.

MONTH: January February March April May June July August September October November December

Day: Monday Tuesday Wednesday Thursday Friday Saturday Sunday
Date: ______ **Season:** Summer Autumn/Fall Winter Spring
Temperature: Low _______ High _______
Barometer: 9am__________ 9pm_________ **Humidity** ____________

Sunny	Cloudy	Rain	Showers	Windy
Snow	Storm	Humid	Dry	

Food & Fluid Intake (be mindful of salt):

Breakfast			
Lunch			
Dinner			
Fluid Intake	Water - ______		
Snacks			

Symptoms:

Tinnitus	Vertigo	Drop Attack	Nausea
Anxiety	Brain Fog	Hearing Loss	Hyperacusis
Fatigue	Balance	Co-ordination	Stress
Headache	Migraine	Nystagmus	Disequilibrium
Ear Fullness/ Pressure/Pain	Vision Difficulties	Physical Impairment	Vestibular Migraine
Vomiting	Depression	BPPV*	Diarrhea
PPPD*	Jaw Click/Pain	Neck Pain	Motion Sensitivity
Sweating	Speech Difficulty	Monthly Cycle	

What time did your symptoms start? ____________________

Tinnitus: L R How many noises? ______ Loudness Scale: 1 2 3 4 5

Possible Meniere's Symptom Triggers Today:

Physical: ____________________

____

____

____________________ Pollen, Mold, Dust, Trees, Grass, Ragweed

Visual: ____________________

____

____

Emotional: ____________________

____

____

What Helped Me?

Medication/s & Time Taken		Other	
		Prayer	Rest
		Meditation	Friend/s
		Self-care	Family
		Exercise	Pet/s
		Mindfulness	Vestibular Rehab
		Gratitude	Hearing Device

Duration of Vertigo ______ minutes ______ hours ______ days

Severity of Vertigo 1 2 3 4 5 - I HATE you, vertigo!

New Symptoms? ____________________

____

What I Accomplished Today – Something to Celebrate! ♡

____

____

____

Three Things I am Thankful for Today:

1.
2.
3.

MONTH: January February March April May June July August September October November December

Day: Monday Tuesday Wednesday Thursday Friday Saturday Sunday
Date: ______ **Season:** Summer Autumn/Fall Winter Spring
Temperature: Low _______ High _______
Barometer: 9am_________ 9pm_________ **Humidity** ___________

Sunny	Cloudy	Rain	Showers	Windy
Snow	Storm	Humid	Dry	

Food & Fluid Intake (be mindful of salt):

Breakfast			
Lunch			
Dinner			
Fluid Intake	Water - ______		
Snacks			

Symptoms:

Tinnitus	Vertigo	Drop Attack	Nausea
Anxiety	Brain Fog	Hearing Loss	Hyperacusis
Fatigue	Balance	Co-ordination	Stress
Headache	Migraine	Nystagmus	Disequilibrium
Ear Fullness/ Pressure/Pain	Vision Difficulties	Physical Impairment	Vestibular Migraine
Vomiting	Depression	BPPV*	Diarrhea
PPPD*	Jaw Click/Pain	Neck Pain	Motion Sensitivity
Sweating	Speech Difficulty	Monthly Cycle	

What time did your symptoms start? ____________________

Tinnitus: L R How many noises? _______ Loudness Scale: 1 2 3 4 5

Possible Meniere's Symptom Triggers Today:

Physical: ____________________

____

____

____________________ Pollen, Mold, Dust, Trees, Grass, Ragweed

Visual: ____________________

____

____

Emotional: ____________________

____

____

What Helped Me?

Medication/s & Time Taken		Other	
		Prayer	Rest
		Meditation	Friend/s
		Self-care	Family
		Exercise	Pet/s
		Mindfulness	Vestibular Rehab
		Gratitude	Hearing Device

Duration of Vertigo ______ minutes ______ hours______ days

Severity of Vertigo 1 2 3 4 5 - I HATE you, vertigo!

New Symptoms? ____________________

____

What I Accomplished Today - Something to Celebrate! ♡

____

____

____

Three Things I am Thankful for Today:

1.
2.
3.

MONTH: January February March April May June July August September October November December

Day: Monday Tuesday Wednesday Thursday Friday Saturday Sunday
Date: ______ **Season:** Summer Autumn/Fall Winter Spring
Temperature: Low ______ High ______
Barometer: 9am______ 9pm______ **Humidity** ______

Sunny	Cloudy	Rain	Showers	Windy
Snow	Storm	Humid	Dry	

Food & Fluid Intake (be mindful of salt):

Breakfast			
Lunch			
Dinner			
Fluid Intake	Water - ______		
Snacks			

Symptoms:

Tinnitus	Vertigo	Drop Attack	Nausea
Anxiety	Brain Fog	Hearing Loss	Hyperacusis
Fatigue	Balance	Co-ordination	Stress
Headache	Migraine	Nystagmus	Disequilibrium
Ear Fullness/ Pressure/Pain	Vision Difficulties	Physical Impairment	Vestibular Migraine
Vomiting	Depression	BPPV*	Diarrhea
PPPD*	Jaw Click/Pain	Neck Pain	Motion Sensitivity
Sweating	Speech Difficulty	Monthly Cycle	

What time did your symptoms start? ____________________

Tinnitus: L R How many noises? _______ Loudness Scale: 1 2 3 4 5

Possible Meniere's Symptom Triggers Today:

Physical: ____________________

____

____

____________________ Pollen, Mold, Dust, Trees, Grass, Ragweed

Visual: ____________________

____

____

Emotional: ____________________

____

____

What Helped Me?

Medication/s & Time Taken		Other	
		Prayer	Rest
		Meditation	Friend/s
		Self-care	Family
		Exercise	Pet/s
		Mindfulness	Vestibular Rehab
		Gratitude	Hearing Device

Duration of Vertigo ______ minutes ______ hours______ days

Severity of Vertigo 1 2 3 4 5 - I HATE you, vertigo!

New Symptoms? ____________________

____

What I Accomplished Today – Something to Celebrate! ♡

____

____

____

Three Things I am Thankful for Today:

1.
2.
3.

MONTH: January February March April May June July August September October November December

Day: Monday Tuesday Wednesday Thursday Friday Saturday Sunday
Date: ______ **Season:** Summer Autumn/Fall Winter Spring
Temperature: Low ______ High ______
Barometer: 9am________ 9pm________ **Humidity** __________

Sunny	Cloudy	Rain	Showers	Windy
Snow	Storm	Humid	Dry	

Food & Fluid Intake (be mindful of salt):

Breakfast			
Lunch			
Dinner			
Fluid Intake	Water - ______		
Snacks			

Symptoms:

Tinnitus	Vertigo	Drop Attack	Nausea
Anxiety	Brain Fog	Hearing Loss	Hyperacusis
Fatigue	Balance	Co-ordination	Stress
Headache	Migraine	Nystagmus	Disequilibrium
Ear Fullness/ Pressure/Pain	Vision Difficulties	Physical Impairment	Vestibular Migraine
Vomiting	Depression	BPPV*	Diarrhea
PPPD*	Jaw Click/Pain	Neck Pain	Motion Sensitivity
Sweating	Speech Difficulty	Monthly Cycle	

What time did your symptoms start? ______________________

Tinnitus: L R How many noises? ______ Loudness Scale: 1 2 3 4 5

Possible Meniere's Symptom Triggers Today:

Physical: ____

____

____

__________________________ Pollen, Mold, Dust, Trees, Grass, Ragweed

Visual: ____

____

____

Emotional: ____

____

____

What Helped Me?

Medication/s & Time Taken		Other	
		Prayer	Rest
		Meditation	Friend/s
		Self-care	Family
		Exercise	Pet/s
		Mindfulness	Vestibular Rehab
		Gratitude	Hearing Device

Duration of Vertigo ______ minutes ______ hours______ days

Severity of Vertigo 1 2 3 4 5 - I HATE you, vertigo!

New Symptoms? ______________________________________

____

What I Accomplished Today - Something to Celebrate! ♡

____

____

____

Three Things I am Thankful for Today:

1.
2.
3.

MONTH: January February March April May June July August September October November December

Day: Monday Tuesday Wednesday Thursday Friday Saturday Sunday
Date: ______ **Season:** Summer Autumn/Fall Winter Spring
Temperature: Low ______ High ______
Barometer: 9am______ 9pm______ **Humidity** __________

Sunny	Cloudy	Rain	Showers	Windy
Snow	Storm	Humid	Dry	

Food & Fluid Intake (be mindful of salt):

Breakfast			
Lunch			
Dinner			
Fluid Intake	Water - ______		
Snacks			

Symptoms:

Tinnitus	Vertigo	Drop Attack	Nausea
Anxiety	Brain Fog	Hearing Loss	Hyperacusis
Fatigue	Balance	Co-ordination	Stress
Headache	Migraine	Nystagmus	Disequilibrium
Ear Fullness/ Pressure/Pain	Vision Difficulties	Physical Impairment	Vestibular Migraine
Vomiting	Depression	BPPV*	Diarrhea
PPPD*	Jaw Click/Pain	Neck Pain	Motion Sensitivity
Sweating	Speech Difficulty	Monthly Cycle	

What time did your symptoms start? ______________

Tinnitus: L R How many noises? _______ Loudness Scale: 1 2 3 4 5

Possible Meniere's Symptom Triggers Today:

Physical: ______________

____

____

______________ Pollen, Mold, Dust, Trees, Grass, Ragweed

Visual: ______________

____

____

Emotional: ______________

____

____

What Helped Me?

Medication/s & Time Taken		Other	
		Prayer	Rest
		Meditation	Friend/s
		Self-care	Family
		Exercise	Pet/s
		Mindfulness	Vestibular Rehab
		Gratitude	Hearing Device

Duration of Vertigo ______ minutes ______ hours ______ days

Severity of Vertigo 1 2 3 4 5 - I HATE you, vertigo!

New Symptoms? ______________

____

What I Accomplished Today – Something to Celebrate! ♡

____

____

____

Three Things I am Thankful for Today:

1.
2.
3.

MONTH: January February March April May June July August September October November December

Day: Monday Tuesday Wednesday Thursday Friday Saturday Sunday
Date: ______ **Season:** Summer Autumn/Fall Winter Spring
Temperature: Low ______ High ______
Barometer: 9am______ 9pm______ **Humidity** ______

Sunny	Cloudy	Rain	Showers	Windy
Snow	Storm	Humid	Dry	

Food & Fluid Intake (be mindful of salt):

Breakfast			
Lunch			
Dinner			
Fluid Intake	Water - ______		
Snacks			

Symptoms:

Tinnitus	Vertigo	Drop Attack	Nausea
Anxiety	Brain Fog	Hearing Loss	Hyperacusis
Fatigue	Balance	Co-ordination	Stress
Headache	Migraine	Nystagmus	Disequilibrium
Ear Fullness/ Pressure/Pain	Vision Difficulties	Physical Impairment	Vestibular Migraine
Vomiting	Depression	BPPV*	Diarrhea
PPPD*	Jaw Click/Pain	Neck Pain	Motion Sensitivity
Sweating	Speech Difficulty	Monthly Cycle	

What time did your symptoms start? ____________________

Tinnitus: L R How many noises? _______ Loudness Scale: 1 2 3 4 5

Possible Meniere's Symptom Triggers Today:

Physical: ____________________

____

____

____________________ Pollen, Mold, Dust, Trees, Grass, Ragweed

Visual: ____________________

____

____

Emotional: ____________________

____

____

What Helped Me?

Medication/s & Time Taken		Other	
		Prayer	Rest
		Meditation	Friend/s
		Self-care	Family
		Exercise	Pet/s
		Mindfulness	Vestibular Rehab
		Gratitude	Hearing Device

Duration of Vertigo ______ minutes ______ hours______ days

Severity of Vertigo 1 2 3 4 5 - I HATE you, vertigo!

New Symptoms? ____________________

____

What I Accomplished Today – Something to Celebrate! ♡

____

____

____

Three Things I am Thankful for Today:

1.
2.
3.

MONTH: January February March April May June July August September October November December

Day: Monday Tuesday Wednesday Thursday Friday Saturday Sunday

Date: ______ **Season:** Summer Autumn/Fall Winter Spring

Temperature: Low _______ High _______

Barometer: 9am_________ 9pm_________ **Humidity** ___________

Sunny	Cloudy	Rain	Showers	Windy
Snow	Storm	Humid	Dry	

Food & Fluid Intake (be mindful of salt):

Breakfast			
Lunch			
Dinner			
Fluid Intake	Water - ______		
Snacks			

Symptoms:

Tinnitus	Vertigo	Drop Attack	Nausea
Anxiety	Brain Fog	Hearing Loss	Hyperacusis
Fatigue	Balance	Co-ordination	Stress
Headache	Migraine	Nystagmus	Disequilibrium
Ear Fullness/ Pressure/Pain	Vision Difficulties	Physical Impairment	Vestibular Migraine
Vomiting	Depression	BPPV*	Diarrhea
PPPD*	Jaw Click/Pain	Neck Pain	Motion Sensitivity
Sweating	Speech Difficulty	Monthly Cycle	

What time did your symptoms start? ____________________

Tinnitus: L R How many noises? _______ Loudness Scale: 1 2 3 4 5

Possible Meniere's Symptom Triggers Today:

Physical: ____________________

____

____

____________________ Pollen, Mold, Dust, Trees, Grass, Ragweed

Visual: ____________________

____

____

Emotional: ____________________

____

____

What Helped Me?

Medication/s & Time Taken		Other	
		Prayer	Rest
		Meditation	Friend/s
		Self-care	Family
		Exercise	Pet/s
		Mindfulness	Vestibular Rehab
		Gratitude	Hearing Device

Duration of Vertigo ______ minutes ______ hours______ days

Severity of Vertigo 1 2 3 4 5 - I HATE you, vertigo!

New Symptoms? ____________________

____

What I Accomplished Today - Something to Celebrate! ♡

____

____

____

Three Things I am Thankful for Today:

1.
2.
3.

MONTH: January February March April May June July August September October November December

Day: Monday Tuesday Wednesday Thursday Friday Saturday Sunday
Date: ______ **Season:** Summer Autumn/Fall Winter Spring
Temperature: Low _______ High _______
Barometer: 9am__________ 9pm__________ **Humidity** ___________

Sunny	Cloudy	Rain	Showers	Windy
Snow	Storm	Humid	Dry	

Food & Fluid Intake (be mindful of salt):

Breakfast			
Lunch			
Dinner			
Fluid Intake	Water - _____		
Snacks			

Symptoms:

Tinnitus	Vertigo	Drop Attack	Nausea
Anxiety	Brain Fog	Hearing Loss	Hyperacusis
Fatigue	Balance	Co-ordination	Stress
Headache	Migraine	Nystagmus	Disequilibrium
Ear Fullness/ Pressure/Pain	Vision Difficulties	Physical Impairment	Vestibular Migraine
Vomiting	Depression	BPPV*	Diarrhea
PPPD*	Jaw Click/Pain	Neck Pain	Motion Sensitivity
Sweating	Speech Difficulty	Monthly Cycle	

What time did your symptoms start? ____________________

Tinnitus: L R How many noises? ______ Loudness Scale: 1 2 3 4 5

Possible Meniere's Symptom Triggers Today:

Physical: ____________________

____

____

____________________ Pollen, Mold, Dust, Trees, Grass, Ragweed

Visual: ____________________

____

Emotional: ____________________

____

____

What Helped Me?

Medication/s & Time Taken		Other	
		Prayer	Rest
		Meditation	Friend/s
		Self-care	Family
		Exercise	Pet/s
		Mindfulness	Vestibular Rehab
		Gratitude	Hearing Device

Duration of Vertigo ______ minutes ______ hours ______ days

Severity of Vertigo 1 2 3 4 5 - I HATE you, vertigo!

New Symptoms? ____________________

____

What I Accomplished Today – Something to Celebrate! ♡

____

____

____

Three Things I am Thankful for Today:

1.
2.
3.

MONTH: January February March April May June July August September October November December

Day: Monday Tuesday Wednesday Thursday Friday Saturday Sunday
Date: ______ **Season:** Summer Autumn/Fall Winter Spring
Temperature: Low _______ High _______
Barometer: 9am_______ 9pm_______ **Humidity** ___________

Sunny	Cloudy	Rain	Showers	Windy
Snow	Storm	Humid	Dry	

Food & Fluid Intake (be mindful of salt):

Breakfast			
Lunch			
Dinner			
Fluid Intake	Water - ____		
Snacks			

Symptoms:

Tinnitus	Vertigo	Drop Attack	Nausea
Anxiety	Brain Fog	Hearing Loss	Hyperacusis
Fatigue	Balance	Co-ordination	Stress
Headache	Migraine	Nystagmus	Disequilibrium
Ear Fullness/ Pressure/Pain	Vision Difficulties	Physical Impairment	Vestibular Migraine
Vomiting	Depression	BPPV*	Diarrhea
PPPD*	Jaw Click/Pain	Neck Pain	Motion Sensitivity
Sweating	Speech Difficulty	Monthly Cycle	

What time did your symptoms start? ____________

Tinnitus: L R How many noises? ______ Loudness Scale: 1 2 3 4 5

Possible Meniere's Symptom Triggers Today:

Physical: ____________

____

____

____________ Pollen, Mold, Dust, Trees, Grass, Ragweed

Visual: ____________

____

____

Emotional: ____________

____

____

What Helped Me?

Medication/s & Time Taken		Other	
		Prayer	Rest
		Meditation	Friend/s
		Self-care	Family
		Exercise	Pet/s
		Mindfulness	Vestibular Rehab
		Gratitude	Hearing Device

Duration of Vertigo ______ minutes ______ hours______ days

Severity of Vertigo 1 2 3 4 5 - I HATE you, vertigo!

New Symptoms? ____________

____

What I Accomplished Today - Something to Celebrate! ♡

____

____

____

Three Things I am Thankful for Today:

1.
2.
3.

MONTH: January February March April May June July August September October November December

Day: Monday Tuesday Wednesday Thursday Friday Saturday Sunday
Date: ______ **Season:** Summer Autumn/Fall Winter Spring
Temperature: Low _______ High _______
Barometer: 9am__________ 9pm__________ **Humidity** ____________

Sunny	Cloudy	Rain	Showers	Windy
Snow	Storm	Humid	Dry	

Food & Fluid Intake (be mindful of salt):

Breakfast			
Lunch			
Dinner			
Fluid Intake	Water -		
Snacks			

Symptoms:

Tinnitus	Vertigo	Drop Attack	Nausea
Anxiety	Brain Fog	Hearing Loss	Hyperacusis
Fatigue	Balance	Co-ordination	Stress
Headache	Migraine	Nystagmus	Disequilibrium
Ear Fullness/ Pressure/Pain	Vision Difficulties	Physical Impairment	Vestibular Migraine
Vomiting	Depression	BPPV*	Diarrhea
PPPD*	Jaw Click/Pain	Neck Pain	Motion Sensitivity
Sweating	Speech Difficulty	Monthly Cycle	

What time did your symptoms start? ______________________

Tinnitus: L R How many noises? ______ Loudness Scale: 1 2 3 4 5

Possible Meniere's Symptom Triggers Today:

Physical: ______________________________________

____

____

______________________ Pollen, Mold, Dust, Trees, Grass, Ragweed

Visual: ______________________________________

____

____

Emotional: ______________________________________

____

____

What Helped Me?

Medication/s & Time Taken		Other	
		Prayer	Rest
		Meditation	Friend/s
		Self-care	Family
		Exercise	Pet/s
		Mindfulness	Vestibular Rehab
		Gratitude	Hearing Device

Duration of Vertigo ______ minutes ______ hours ______ days

Severity of Vertigo 1 2 3 4 5 - I HATE you, vertigo!

New Symptoms? ______________________________________

____

What I Accomplished Today – Something to Celebrate! ♡

____

____

____

Three Things I am Thankful for Today:

1.
2.
3.

MONTH: January February March April May June July August September October November December

Day: Monday Tuesday Wednesday Thursday Friday Saturday Sunday
Date: ______ **Season:** Summer Autumn/Fall Winter Spring
Temperature: Low ______ High ______
Barometer: 9am ______ 9pm ______ **Humidity** ______

Sunny	Cloudy	Rain	Showers	Windy
Snow	Storm	Humid	Dry	

Food & Fluid Intake (be mindful of salt):

Breakfast			
Lunch			
Dinner			
Fluid Intake	Water - ______		
Snacks			

Symptoms:

Tinnitus	Vertigo	Drop Attack	Nausea
Anxiety	Brain Fog	Hearing Loss	Hyperacusis
Fatigue	Balance	Co-ordination	Stress
Headache	Migraine	Nystagmus	Disequilibrium
Ear Fullness/ Pressure/Pain	Vision Difficulties	Physical Impairment	Vestibular Migraine
Vomiting	Depression	BPPV*	Diarrhea
PPPD*	Jaw Click/Pain	Neck Pain	Motion Sensitivity
Sweating	Speech Difficulty	Monthly Cycle	

What time did your symptoms start? ____________________

Tinnitus: L R How many noises? ______ Loudness Scale: 1 2 3 4 5

Possible Meniere's Symptom Triggers Today:

Physical: ____________________

____

____

____________________ Pollen, Mold, Dust, Trees, Grass, Ragweed

Visual: ____________________

____

____

Emotional: ____________________

____

____

What Helped Me?

Medication/s & Time Taken		Other	
		Prayer	Rest
		Meditation	Friend/s
		Self-care	Family
		Exercise	Pet/s
		Mindfulness	Vestibular Rehab
		Gratitude	Hearing Device

Duration of Vertigo ______ minutes ______ hours______ days

Severity of Vertigo 1 2 3 4 5 - I HATE you, vertigo!

New Symptoms? ____________________

____

What I Accomplished Today – Something to Celebrate! ♡

____

____

____

Three Things I am Thankful for Today:

1.
2.
3.

MONTH: January February March April May June July August September October November December

Day: Monday Tuesday Wednesday Thursday Friday Saturday Sunday
Date: ______ **Season:** Summer Autumn/Fall Winter Spring
Temperature: Low ______ High ______
Barometer: 9am______ 9pm______ **Humidity** ______

Sunny	Cloudy	Rain	Showers	Windy
Snow	Storm	Humid	Dry	

Food & Fluid Intake (be mindful of salt):

Breakfast			
Lunch			
Dinner			
Fluid Intake	Water - ______		
Snacks			

Symptoms:

Tinnitus	Vertigo	Drop Attack	Nausea
Anxiety	Brain Fog	Hearing Loss	Hyperacusis
Fatigue	Balance	Co-ordination	Stress
Headache	Migraine	Nystagmus	Disequilibrium
Ear Fullness/ Pressure/Pain	Vision Difficulties	Physical Impairment	Vestibular Migraine
Vomiting	Depression	BPPV*	Diarrhea
PPPD*	Jaw Click/Pain	Neck Pain	Motion Sensitivity
Sweating	Speech Difficulty	Monthly Cycle	

What time did your symptoms start? ______________________

Tinnitus: L R How many noises? ________ Loudness Scale: 1 2 3 4 5

Possible Meniere's Symptom Triggers Today:

Physical: ____

____

____

______________________ Pollen, Mold, Dust, Trees, Grass, Ragweed

Visual: ____

____

____

Emotional: ____

____

____

What Helped Me?

Medication/s & Time Taken		Other	
		Prayer	Rest
		Meditation	Friend/s
		Self-care	Family
		Exercise	Pet/s
		Mindfulness	Vestibular Rehab
		Gratitude	Hearing Device

Duration of Vertigo _______ minutes ________ hours______ days

Severity of Vertigo 1 2 3 4 5 - I HATE you, vertigo!

New Symptoms? ____

____

What I Accomplished Today - Something to Celebrate! ♡

____

____

____

Three Things I am Thankful for Today:

1.
2.
3.

MONTH: January February March April May June July August September October November December

Day: Monday Tuesday Wednesday Thursday Friday Saturday Sunday

Date: _______ **Season:** Summer Autumn/Fall Winter Spring

Temperature: Low ________ High ________

Barometer: 9am__________ 9pm_________ **Humidity** ____________

Sunny	Cloudy	Rain	Showers	Windy
Snow	Storm	Humid	Dry	

Food & Fluid Intake (be mindful of salt):

Breakfast			
Lunch			
Dinner			
Fluid Intake	Water - _______		
Snacks			

Symptoms:

Tinnitus	Vertigo	Drop Attack	Nausea
Anxiety	Brain Fog	Hearing Loss	Hyperacusis
Fatigue	Balance	Co-ordination	Stress
Headache	Migraine	Nystagmus	Disequilibrium
Ear Fullness/ Pressure/Pain	Vision Difficulties	Physical Impairment	Vestibular Migraine
Vomiting	Depression	BPPV*	Diarrhea
PPPD*	Jaw Click/Pain	Neck Pain	Motion Sensitivity
Sweating	Speech Difficulty	Monthly Cycle	

What time did your symptoms start? ______________________

Tinnitus: L R How many noises? _______ Loudness Scale: 1 2 3 4 5

Possible Meniere's Symptom Triggers Today:

Physical: ____

____

____

______________________ Pollen, Mold, Dust, Trees, Grass, Ragweed

Visual: ____

____

____

Emotional: ____

____

____

What Helped Me?

Medication/s & Time Taken		Other	
		Prayer	Rest
		Meditation	Friend/s
		Self-care	Family
		Exercise	Pet/s
		Mindfulness	Vestibular Rehab
		Gratitude	Hearing Device

Duration of Vertigo ______ minutes ______ hours ______ days

Severity of Vertigo 1 2 3 4 5 - I HATE you, vertigo!

New Symptoms? ____

____

What I Accomplished Today – Something to Celebrate! ♡

____

____

____

Three Things I am Thankful for Today:

1.
2.
3.

MONTH: January February March April May June July August September October November December

Day: Monday Tuesday Wednesday Thursday Friday Saturday Sunday
Date: ______ **Season:** Summer Autumn/Fall Winter Spring
Temperature: Low ______ High ______
Barometer: 9am______ 9pm______ **Humidity** ______

Sunny	Cloudy	Rain	Showers	Windy
Snow	Storm	Humid	Dry	

Food & Fluid Intake (be mindful of salt):

Breakfast			
Lunch			
Dinner			
Fluid Intake	Water - ______		
Snacks			

Symptoms:

Tinnitus	Vertigo	Drop Attack	Nausea
Anxiety	Brain Fog	Hearing Loss	Hyperacusis
Fatigue	Balance	Co-ordination	Stress
Headache	Migraine	Nystagmus	Disequilibrium
Ear Fullness/ Pressure/Pain	Vision Difficulties	Physical Impairment	Vestibular Migraine
Vomiting	Depression	BPPV*	Diarrhea
PPPD*	Jaw Click/Pain	Neck Pain	Motion Sensitivity
Sweating	Speech Difficulty	Monthly Cycle	

What time did your symptoms start? ____________________

Tinnitus: L R How many noises? ______ Loudness Scale: 1 2 3 4 5

Possible Meniere's Symptom Triggers Today:

Physical: ____________________

____

____

____________________ Pollen, Mold, Dust, Trees, Grass, Ragweed

Visual: ____________________

____

____

Emotional: ____________________

____

____

What Helped Me?

Medication/s & Time Taken		Other	
		Prayer	Rest
		Meditation	Friend/s
		Self-care	Family
		Exercise	Pet/s
		Mindfulness	Vestibular Rehab
		Gratitude	Hearing Device

Duration of Vertigo ______ minutes ______ hours______ days

Severity of Vertigo 1 2 3 4 5 - I HATE you, vertigo!

New Symptoms? ____________________

____

What I Accomplished Today - Something to Celebrate! ♡

____

____

____

Three Things I am Thankful for Today:

1.
2.
3.

MONTH: January February March April May June July August September October November December

Day: Monday Tuesday Wednesday Thursday Friday Saturday Sunday
Date: ______ **Season:** Summer Autumn/Fall Winter Spring
Temperature: Low _______ High _______
Barometer: 9am__________ 9pm__________ **Humidity** ____________

Sunny	Cloudy	Rain	Showers	Windy
Snow	Storm	Humid	Dry	

Food & Fluid Intake (be mindful of salt):

Breakfast			
Lunch			
Dinner			
Fluid Intake	Water - _______		
Snacks			

Symptoms:

Tinnitus	Vertigo	Drop Attack	Nausea
Anxiety	Brain Fog	Hearing Loss	Hyperacusis
Fatigue	Balance	Co-ordination	Stress
Headache	Migraine	Nystagmus	Disequilibrium
Ear Fullness/ Pressure/Pain	Vision Difficulties	Physical Impairment	Vestibular Migraine
Vomiting	Depression	BPPV*	Diarrhea
PPPD*	Jaw Click/Pain	Neck Pain	Motion Sensitivity
Sweating	Speech Difficulty	Monthly Cycle	

What time did your symptoms start? ______________________

Tinnitus: L R How many noises? ________ Loudness Scale: 1 2 3 4 5

Possible Meniere's Symptom Triggers Today:

Physical: ____

____

____

______________________ Pollen, Mold, Dust, Trees, Grass, Ragweed

Visual: ____

____

____

Emotional: ____

____

____

What Helped Me?

Medication/s & Time Taken		Other	
		Prayer	Rest
		Meditation	Friend/s
		Self-care	Family
		Exercise	Pet/s
		Mindfulness	Vestibular Rehab
		Gratitude	Hearing Device

Duration of Vertigo ______ minutes ______ hours ______ days

Severity of Vertigo 1 2 3 4 5 - I HATE you, vertigo!

New Symptoms? ____

____

What I Accomplished Today - Something to Celebrate! ♡

____

____

____

Three Things I am Thankful for Today:

1.
2.
3.

MONTH: January February March April May June July August September October November December

Day: Monday Tuesday Wednesday Thursday Friday Saturday Sunday
Date: ______ **Season:** Summer Autumn/Fall Winter Spring
Temperature: Low _______ High _______
Barometer: 9am_________ 9pm________ **Humidity** ____________

Sunny	Cloudy	Rain	Showers	Windy
Snow	Storm	Humid	Dry	

Food & Fluid Intake (be mindful of salt):

Breakfast			
Lunch			
Dinner			
Fluid Intake	Water - ______		
Snacks			

Symptoms:

Tinnitus	Vertigo	Drop Attack	Nausea
Anxiety	Brain Fog	Hearing Loss	Hyperacusis
Fatigue	Balance	Co-ordination	Stress
Headache	Migraine	Nystagmus	Disequilibrium
Ear Fullness/ Pressure/Pain	Vision Difficulties	Physical Impairment	Vestibular Migraine
Vomiting	Depression	BPPV*	Diarrhea
PPPD*	Jaw Click/Pain	Neck Pain	Motion Sensitivity
Sweating	Speech Difficulty	Monthly Cycle	

What time did your symptoms start? ____________________

Tinnitus: L R How many noises? ______ Loudness Scale: 1 2 3 4 5

Possible Meniere's Symptom Triggers Today:

Physical: ____________________

____

____

____________________ Pollen, Mold, Dust, Trees, Grass, Ragweed

Visual: ____________________

____

____

Emotional: ____________________

____

____

What Helped Me?

Medication/s & Time Taken		Other	
		Prayer	Rest
		Meditation	Friend/s
		Self-care	Family
		Exercise	Pet/s
		Mindfulness	Vestibular Rehab
		Gratitude	Hearing Device

Duration of Vertigo ______ minutes ______ hours ______ days

Severity of Vertigo 1 2 3 4 5 - I HATE you, vertigo!

New Symptoms? ____________________

____

What I Accomplished Today – Something to Celebrate! ♡

____

____

____

Three Things I am Thankful for Today:

1.
2.
3.

MONTH: January February March April May June July August September October November December

Day: Monday Tuesday Wednesday Thursday Friday Saturday Sunday
Date: ______ **Season:** Summer Autumn/Fall Winter Spring
Temperature: Low _______ High _______
Barometer: 9am_________ 9pm_________ **Humidity** ___________

Sunny	Cloudy	Rain	Showers	Windy
Snow	Storm	Humid	Dry	

Food & Fluid Intake (be mindful of salt):

Breakfast			
Lunch			
Dinner			
Fluid Intake	Water -		
Snacks			

Symptoms:

Tinnitus	Vertigo	Drop Attack	Nausea
Anxiety	Brain Fog	Hearing Loss	Hyperacusis
Fatigue	Balance	Co-ordination	Stress
Headache	Migraine	Nystagmus	Disequilibrium
Ear Fullness/ Pressure/Pain	Vision Difficulties	Physical Impairment	Vestibular Migraine
Vomiting	Depression	BPPV*	Diarrhea
PPPD*	Jaw Click/Pain	Neck Pain	Motion Sensitivity
Sweating	Speech Difficulty	Monthly Cycle	

What time did your symptoms start? ____________________

Tinnitus: L R How many noises? ______ Loudness Scale: 1 2 3 4 5

Possible Meniere's Symptom Triggers Today:

Physical: ____________________

____

____

____________________ Pollen, Mold, Dust, Trees, Grass, Ragweed

Visual: ____________________

____

____

Emotional: ____________________

____

____

What Helped Me?

Medication/s & Time Taken		Other	
		Prayer	Rest
		Meditation	Friend/s
		Self-care	Family
		Exercise	Pet/s
		Mindfulness	Vestibular Rehab
		Gratitude	Hearing Device

Duration of Vertigo ______ minutes ______ hours ______ days

Severity of Vertigo 1 2 3 4 5 - I HATE you, vertigo!

New Symptoms? ____________________

____

What I Accomplished Today - Something to Celebrate! ♡

____

____

____

Three Things I am Thankful for Today:

1.
2.
3.

MONTH: January February March April May June July August September October November December

Day: Monday Tuesday Wednesday Thursday Friday Saturday Sunday
Date: ______ **Season:** Summer Autumn/Fall Winter Spring
Temperature: Low ______ High ______
Barometer: 9am______ 9pm______ **Humidity** ______

Sunny	Cloudy	Rain	Showers	Windy
Snow	Storm	Humid	Dry	

Food & Fluid Intake (be mindful of salt):

Breakfast			
Lunch			
Dinner			
Fluid Intake	Water - ______		
Snacks			

Symptoms:

Tinnitus	Vertigo	Drop Attack	Nausea
Anxiety	Brain Fog	Hearing Loss	Hyperacusis
Fatigue	Balance	Co-ordination	Stress
Headache	Migraine	Nystagmus	Disequilibrium
Ear Fullness/ Pressure/Pain	Vision Difficulties	Physical Impairment	Vestibular Migraine
Vomiting	Depression	BPPV*	Diarrhea
PPPD*	Jaw Click/Pain	Neck Pain	Motion Sensitivity
Sweating	Speech Difficulty	Monthly Cycle	

What time did your symptoms start? ____________________

Tinnitus: L R How many noises? ______ Loudness Scale: 1 2 3 4 5

Possible Meniere's Symptom Triggers Today:

Physical: ____________________

____

____

____________________ Pollen, Mold, Dust, Trees, Grass, Ragweed

Visual: ____________________

____

____

Emotional: ____________________

____

____

What Helped Me?

Medication/s & Time Taken		Other	
		Prayer	Rest
		Meditation	Friend/s
		Self-care	Family
		Exercise	Pet/s
		Mindfulness	Vestibular Rehab
		Gratitude	Hearing Device

Duration of Vertigo ______ minutes ______ hours______ days

Severity of Vertigo 1 2 3 4 5 - I HATE you, vertigo!

New Symptoms? ____________________

____

What I Accomplished Today – Something to Celebrate! ♡

____

____

____

Three Things I am Thankful for Today:

1.
2.
3.

Vertigo. STOP! There will be a cure! Meniere's disease does not define us. Meniere's, I hate you! Tinnitus. MENIERE'S WARRIOR! Hope – there is always hope! Hearing loss. A cure will be found! Imbalance. Take each day one at a time. BREATHE. Create moments. Find things to be thankful for. Ear pain. You will overcome. Good things are coming. Research. Meniere's, your time is UP! Vertigo. There will be a cure! Meniere's disease does not define us. Meniere's, I hate you! Tinnitus. MENIERE'S WARRIOR! Hope – there is always hope! Hearing loss. A cure will be found! Imbalance. Take each day one at a time. BREATHE. Create moments. Find things to be thankful for. Ear pain. You will overcome. Good things are coming. Research. Meniere's, your time is UP! Vertigo. There will be a cure! Meniere's disease does not define us. Meniere's, I hate you! Tinnitus. MENIERE'S WARRIOR! Hope – there is always hope! Hearing loss. A cure will be found! Imbalance. Take each day one at a time. BREATHE. Create moments. Find things to be thankful for. Ear pain. You will overcome. Good things are coming. Research. Meniere's, your time is UP! Vertigo. There will be a cure! Meniere's disease does not define us. Meniere's, I hate you! Tinnitus. MENIERE'S WARRIOR! Hope, there is always hope! We will be cured! BREATHE...vertigo. STOP! There will be a cure! Meniere's disease does not define us. Meniere's, I hate you! Tinnitus. MENIERE'S WARRIOR! Hope – there is always hope! Hearing loss. A cure will be found! Imbalance. Take each day one at a time. BREATHE. Create moments. Find things to be thankful for. Ear pain. You will overcome. Good things are coming. Research. Meniere's, your time is UP! Vertigo. There will be a cure! Meniere's disease does not define us. Meniere's, I hate you! Tinnitus. MENIERE'S WARRIOR! Hope – there is always hope! Hearing loss. A cure will be found! Imbalance. Take each day one at a time. BREATHE. Create moments. Find things to be thankful for. Ear pain. You will overcome. Good things are coming. Research. Meniere's, your time is UP! Vertigo. There will be a cure! Meniere's disease does not define us. Meniere's, I hate you! Tinnitus. MENIERE'S WARRIOR! Hope – there is always hope! Hearing loss. A cure will be found! Imbalance. Take each day one at a time. BREATHE. Create moments. Find things to be thankful for. Ear pain. You will overcome. Good things are coming. Research. Meniere's, your time is UP! Vertigo. There will be a cure! Meniere's disease does not define us. Meniere's, I hate you! Tinnitus. MENIERE'S WARRIOR! Hope, there is always hope! We will be cured! BREATHE...vertigo. STOP! There will be a cure! Meniere's disease does not define us. Meniere's, I hate you! Tinnitus. MENIERE'S WARRIOR! Hope – there is always hope! Hearing loss. A cure will be found! Imbalance. Take each day one at a time. BREATHE. Create moments. Find things to be thankful for. Ear pain. You will overcome. Good things are coming. Research. Meniere's, your time is UP! Vertigo. **There will be a cure!**

Vertigo. STOP! There will be a cure! Meniere's disease does not define us. Meniere's, I hate you! Tinnitus. MENIERE'S WARRIOR! Hope – there is always hope! Hearing loss. A cure will be found! Imbalance. Take each day one at a time. BREATHE. Create moments. Find things to be thankful for. Ear pain. You will overcome. Good things are coming. Research. Meniere's, your time is UP! Vertigo. There will be a cure! Meniere's disease does not define us. Meniere's, I hate you! Tinnitus. MENIERE'S WARRIOR! Hope – there is always hope! Hearing loss. A cure will be found! Imbalance. Take each day one at a time. BREATHE. Create moments. Find things to be thankful for. Ear pain. You will overcome. Good things are coming. Research. Meniere's, your time is UP! Vertigo. There will be a cure! Meniere's disease does not define us. Meniere's, I hate you! Tinnitus. MENIERE'S WARRIOR! Hope – there is always hope! Hearing loss. A cure will be found! Imbalance. Take each day one at a time. BREATHE. Create moments. Find things to be thankful for. Ear pain. You will overcome. Good things are coming. Research. Meniere's, your time is UP! Vertigo. There will be a cure! Meniere's disease does not define us. Meniere's, I hate you! Tinnitus. MENIERE'S WARRIOR! Hope, there is always hope! We will be cured! BREATHE...vertigo. STOP! There will be a cure! Meniere's disease does not define us. Meniere's, I hate you! Tinnitus. MENIERE'S WARRIOR! Hope – there is always hope! Hearing loss. A cure will be found! Imbalance. Take each day one at a time. BREATHE. Create moments. Find things to be thankful for. Ear pain. You will overcome. Good things are coming. Research. Meniere's, your time is UP! Vertigo. There will be a cure! Meniere's disease does not define us. Meniere's, I hate you! Tinnitus. MENIERE'S WARRIOR! Hope – there is always hope! Hearing loss. A cure will be found! Imbalance. Take each day one at a time. BREATHE. Create moments. Find things to be thankful for. Ear pain. You will overcome. Good things are coming. Research. Meniere's, your time is UP! Vertigo. There will be a cure! Meniere's disease does not define us. Meniere's, I hate you! Tinnitus. MENIERE'S WARRIOR! Hope – there is always hope! Hearing loss. A cure will be found! Imbalance. Take each day one at a time. BREATHE. Create moments. Find things to be thankful for. Ear pain. You will overcome. Good things are coming. Research. Meniere's, your time is UP! Vertigo. There will be a cure! Meniere's disease does not define us. Meniere's, I hate you! Tinnitus. MENIERE'S WARRIOR! Hope, there is always hope! We will be cured! BREATHE...vertigo. STOP! There will be a cure! Meniere's disease does not define us. Meniere's, I hate you! Tinnitus. MENIERE'S WARRIOR! Hope – there is always hope! Hearing loss. A cure will be found! Imbalance. Take each day one at a time. BREATHE. Create moments. Find things to be thankful for. Ear pain. You will overcome. Good things are coming. Research. Meniere's, your time is UP! Vertigo. **There will be a cure!**

MONTH: January February March April May June July August September October November December

Day: Monday Tuesday Wednesday Thursday Friday Saturday Sunday
Date: ______ **Season:** Summer Autumn/Fall Winter Spring
Temperature: Low ______ High ______
Barometer: 9am__________ 9pm__________ **Humidity** __________

Sunny	Cloudy	Rain	Showers	Windy
Snow	Storm	Humid	Dry	

Food & Fluid Intake (be mindful of salt):

Breakfast			
Lunch			
Dinner			
Fluid Intake	Water - ______		
Snacks			

Symptoms:

Tinnitus	Vertigo	Drop Attack	Nausea
Anxiety	Brain Fog	Hearing Loss	Hyperacusis
Fatigue	Balance	Co-ordination	Stress
Headache	Migraine	Nystagmus	Disequilibrium
Ear Fullness/ Pressure/Pain	Vision Difficulties	Physical Impairment	Vestibular Migraine
Vomiting	Depression	BPPV*	Diarrhea
PPPD*	Jaw Click/Pain	Neck Pain	Motion Sensitivity
Sweating	Speech Difficulty	Monthly Cycle	

What time did your symptoms start? ____________________

Tinnitus: L R How many noises? ______ Loudness Scale: 1 2 3 4 5

Possible Meniere's Symptom Triggers Today:

Physical: ____________________

____

____

____________________ Pollen, Mold, Dust, Trees, Grass, Ragweed

Visual: ____________________

____

____

Emotional: ____________________

____

____

What Helped Me?

Medication/s & Time Taken		Other	
		Prayer	Rest
		Meditation	Friend/s
		Self-care	Family
		Exercise	Pet/s
		Mindfulness	Vestibular Rehab
		Gratitude	Hearing Device

Duration of Vertigo ______ minutes ______ hours ______ days

Severity of Vertigo 1 2 3 4 5 - I HATE you, vertigo!

New Symptoms? ____________________

____

What I Accomplished Today – Something to Celebrate! ♡

____

____

____

Three Things I am Thankful for Today:

1.
2.
3.

MONTH: January February March April May June July August September October November December

Day: Monday Tuesday Wednesday Thursday Friday Saturday Sunday
Date: ______ **Season:** Summer Autumn/Fall Winter Spring
Temperature: Low ______ High ______
Barometer: 9am______ 9pm______ **Humidity** ______

Sunny	Cloudy	Rain	Showers	Windy
Snow	Storm	Humid	Dry	

Food & Fluid Intake (be mindful of salt):

Breakfast			
Lunch			
Dinner			
Fluid Intake	Water - ______		
Snacks			

Symptoms:

Tinnitus	Vertigo	Drop Attack	Nausea
Anxiety	Brain Fog	Hearing Loss	Hyperacusis
Fatigue	Balance	Co-ordination	Stress
Headache	Migraine	Nystagmus	Disequilibrium
Ear Fullness/ Pressure/Pain	Vision Difficulties	Physical Impairment	Vestibular Migraine
Vomiting	Depression	BPPV*	Diarrhea
PPPD*	Jaw Click/Pain	Neck Pain	Motion Sensitivity
Sweating	Speech Difficulty	Monthly Cycle	

What time did your symptoms start? ______________________

Tinnitus: L R How many noises? ________ Loudness Scale: 1 2 3 4 5

Possible Meniere's Symptom Triggers Today:

Physical: ______________________

____

____

______________________ Pollen, Mold, Dust, Trees, Grass, Ragweed

Visual: ______________________

____

____

Emotional: ______________________

____

____

What Helped Me?

Medication/s & Time Taken		Other	
		Prayer	Rest
		Meditation	Friend/s
		Self-care	Family
		Exercise	Pet/s
		Mindfulness	Vestibular Rehab
		Gratitude	Hearing Device

Duration of Vertigo ______ minutes ______ hours______ days

Severity of Vertigo 1 2 3 4 5 - I HATE you, vertigo!

New Symptoms? ______________________

____

What I Accomplished Today - Something to Celebrate! ♡

____

____

____

Three Things I am Thankful for Today:

1.
2.
3.

MONTH: January February March April May June July August September October November December

Day: Monday Tuesday Wednesday Thursday Friday Saturday Sunday
Date: ______ **Season:** Summer Autumn/Fall Winter Spring
Temperature: Low ______ High ______
Barometer: 9am________ 9pm________ **Humidity** __________

Sunny	Cloudy	Rain	Showers	Windy
Snow	Storm	Humid	Dry	

Food & Fluid Intake (be mindful of salt):

Breakfast			
Lunch			
Dinner			
Fluid Intake	Water - ______		
Snacks			

Symptoms:

Tinnitus	Vertigo	Drop Attack	Nausea
Anxiety	Brain Fog	Hearing Loss	Hyperacusis
Fatigue	Balance	Co-ordination	Stress
Headache	Migraine	Nystagmus	Disequilibrium
Ear Fullness/ Pressure/Pain	Vision Difficulties	Physical Impairment	Vestibular Migraine
Vomiting	Depression	BPPV*	Diarrhea
PPPD*	Jaw Click/Pain	Neck Pain	Motion Sensitivity
Sweating	Speech Difficulty	Monthly Cycle	

What time did your symptoms start? ______________________

Tinnitus: L R How many noises? ______ Loudness Scale: 1 2 3 4 5

Possible Meniere's Symptom Triggers Today:

Physical: ____

____

____

______________________ Pollen, Mold, Dust, Trees, Grass, Ragweed

Visual: ____

____

Emotional: ____

____

____

What Helped Me?

Medication/s & Time Taken		Other	
		Prayer	Rest
		Meditation	Friend/s
		Self-care	Family
		Exercise	Pet/s
		Mindfulness	Vestibular Rehab
		Gratitude	Hearing Device

Duration of Vertigo ______ minutes ______ hours______ days

Severity of Vertigo 1 2 3 4 5 - I HATE you, vertigo!

New Symptoms? ____

____

What I Accomplished Today - Something to Celebrate! ♡

____

____

____

Three Things I am Thankful for Today:

1.
2.
3.

MONTH: January February March April May June July August September October November December

Day: Monday Tuesday Wednesday Thursday Friday Saturday Sunday
Date: ______ **Season:** Summer Autumn/Fall Winter Spring
Temperature: Low _______ High _______
Barometer: 9am_________ 9pm_________ **Humidity** ___________

Sunny	Cloudy	Rain	Showers	Windy
Snow	Storm	Humid	Dry	

Food & Fluid Intake (be mindful of salt):

Breakfast			
Lunch			
Dinner			
Fluid Intake	Water - ______		
Snacks			

Symptoms:

Tinnitus	Vertigo	Drop Attack	Nausea
Anxiety	Brain Fog	Hearing Loss	Hyperacusis
Fatigue	Balance	Co-ordination	Stress
Headache	Migraine	Nystagmus	Disequilibrium
Ear Fullness/ Pressure/Pain	Vision Difficulties	Physical Impairment	Vestibular Migraine
Vomiting	Depression	BPPV*	Diarrhea
PPPD*	Jaw Click/Pain	Neck Pain	Motion Sensitivity
Sweating	Speech Difficulty	Monthly Cycle	

What time did your symptoms start? ______________________

Tinnitus: L R How many noises? ______ Loudness Scale: 1 2 3 4 5

Possible Meniere's Symptom Triggers Today:

Physical: ____

____

____

______________________ Pollen, Mold, Dust, Trees, Grass, Ragweed

Visual: ____

____

____

Emotional: ____

____

____

What Helped Me?

Medication/s & Time Taken		Other	
		Prayer	Rest
		Meditation	Friend/s
		Self-care	Family
		Exercise	Pet/s
		Mindfulness	Vestibular Rehab
		Gratitude	Hearing Device

Duration of Vertigo ______ minutes ______ hours ______ days

Severity of Vertigo 1 2 3 4 5 - I HATE you, vertigo!

New Symptoms? ____

____

What I Accomplished Today - Something to Celebrate! ♡

____

____

____

Three Things I am Thankful for Today:

1.
2.
3.

MONTH: January February March April May June July August September October November December

Day: Monday Tuesday Wednesday Thursday Friday Saturday Sunday

Date: ______ **Season:** Summer Autumn/Fall Winter Spring

Temperature: Low ______ High ______

Barometer: 9am______ 9pm______ **Humidity** ______

Sunny	Cloudy	Rain	Showers	Windy
Snow	Storm	Humid	Dry	

Food & Fluid Intake (be mindful of salt):

Breakfast			
Lunch			
Dinner			
Fluid Intake	Water - ______		
Snacks			

Symptoms:

Tinnitus	Vertigo	Drop Attack	Nausea
Anxiety	Brain Fog	Hearing Loss	Hyperacusis
Fatigue	Balance	Co-ordination	Stress
Headache	Migraine	Nystagmus	Disequilibrium
Ear Fullness/ Pressure/Pain	Vision Difficulties	Physical Impairment	Vestibular Migraine
Vomiting	Depression	BPPV*	Diarrhea
PPPD*	Jaw Click/Pain	Neck Pain	Motion Sensitivity
Sweating	Speech Difficulty	Monthly Cycle	

What time did your symptoms start? ____________________

Tinnitus: L R How many noises? ________ Loudness Scale: 1 2 3 4 5

Possible Meniere's Symptom Triggers Today:

Physical: ____________________

____

____

____________________ Pollen, Mold, Dust, Trees, Grass, Ragweed

Visual: ____________________

____

____

Emotional: ____________________

____

____

What Helped Me?

Medication/s & Time Taken		Other	
		Prayer	Rest
		Meditation	Friend/s
		Self-care	Family
		Exercise	Pet/s
		Mindfulness	Vestibular Rehab
		Gratitude	Hearing Device

Duration of Vertigo ______ minutes ______ hours______ days

Severity of Vertigo 1 2 3 4 5 - I HATE you, vertigo!

New Symptoms? ____________________

____

What I Accomplished Today - Something to Celebrate! ♡

____

____

____

Three Things I am Thankful for Today:

1.
2.
3.

MONTH: January February March April May June July August September October November December

Day: Monday Tuesday Wednesday Thursday Friday Saturday Sunday

Date: ______ **Season:** Summer Autumn/Fall Winter Spring

Temperature: Low _______ High _______

Barometer: 9am_________ 9pm________ **Humidity** ____________

Sunny	Cloudy	Rain	Showers	Windy
Snow	Storm	Humid	Dry	

Food & Fluid Intake (be mindful of salt):

Breakfast			
Lunch			
Dinner			
Fluid Intake	Water - ______		
Snacks			

Symptoms:

Tinnitus	Vertigo	Drop Attack	Nausea
Anxiety	Brain Fog	Hearing Loss	Hyperacusis
Fatigue	Balance	Co-ordination	Stress
Headache	Migraine	Nystagmus	Disequilibrium
Ear Fullness/ Pressure/Pain	Vision Difficulties	Physical Impairment	Vestibular Migraine
Vomiting	Depression	BPPV*	Diarrhea
PPPD*	Jaw Click/Pain	Neck Pain	Motion Sensitivity
Sweating	Speech Difficulty	Monthly Cycle	

What time did your symptoms start? ___________________

Tinnitus: L R How many noises? ______ Loudness Scale: 1 2 3 4 5

Possible Meniere's Symptom Triggers Today:

Physical: ___________________

____

____

___________________ Pollen, Mold, Dust, Trees, Grass, Ragweed

Visual: ___________________

____

Emotional: ___________________

____

____

What Helped Me?

Medication/s & Time Taken		Other	
		Prayer	Rest
		Meditation	Friend/s
		Self-care	Family
		Exercise	Pet/s
		Mindfulness	Vestibular Rehab
		Gratitude	Hearing Device

Duration of Vertigo ______ minutes ______ hours ______ days

Severity of Vertigo 1 2 3 4 5 - I HATE you, vertigo!

New Symptoms? ___________________

____

What I Accomplished Today - Something to Celebrate! ♡

____

____

____

Three Things I am Thankful for Today:

1.
2.
3.

MONTH: January February March April May June July August September October November December

Day: Monday Tuesday Wednesday Thursday Friday Saturday Sunday
Date: ______ **Season:** Summer Autumn/Fall Winter Spring
Temperature: Low _______ High _______
Barometer: 9am__________ 9pm__________ **Humidity** __________

Sunny	Cloudy	Rain	Showers	Windy
Snow	Storm	Humid	Dry	

Food & Fluid Intake (be mindful of salt):

Breakfast			
Lunch			
Dinner			
Fluid Intake	Water - ____		
Snacks			

Symptoms:

Tinnitus	Vertigo	Drop Attack	Nausea
Anxiety	Brain Fog	Hearing Loss	Hyperacusis
Fatigue	Balance	Co-ordination	Stress
Headache	Migraine	Nystagmus	Disequilibrium
Ear Fullness/ Pressure/Pain	Vision Difficulties	Physical Impairment	Vestibular Migraine
Vomiting	Depression	BPPV*	Diarrhea
PPPD*	Jaw Click/Pain	Neck Pain	Motion Sensitivity
Sweating	Speech Difficulty	Monthly Cycle	

What time did your symptoms start? ____________________

Tinnitus: L R How many noises? ______ Loudness Scale: 1 2 3 4 5

Possible Meniere's Symptom Triggers Today:

Physical: ____________________

____

____

____________________ Pollen, Mold, Dust, Trees, Grass, Ragweed

Visual: ____________________

____

____

Emotional: ____________________

____

____

What Helped Me?

Medication/s & Time Taken		Other	
		Prayer	Rest
		Meditation	Friend/s
		Self-care	Family
		Exercise	Pet/s
		Mindfulness	Vestibular Rehab
		Gratitude	Hearing Device

Duration of Vertigo ______ minutes ______ hours______ days

Severity of Vertigo 1 2 3 4 5 - I HATE you, vertigo!

New Symptoms? ____________________

____

What I Accomplished Today - Something to Celebrate! ♡

____

____

____

Three Things I am Thankful for Today:

1.
2.
3.

MONTH: January February March April May June July August September October November December

Day: Monday Tuesday Wednesday Thursday Friday Saturday Sunday

Date: ______ **Season:** Summer Autumn/Fall Winter Spring

Temperature: Low _______ High _______

Barometer: 9am__________ 9pm__________ **Humidity** ____________

Sunny	Cloudy	Rain	Showers	Windy
Snow	Storm	Humid	Dry	

Food & Fluid Intake (be mindful of salt):

Breakfast			
Lunch			
Dinner			
Fluid Intake	Water - ______		
Snacks			

Symptoms:

Tinnitus	Vertigo	Drop Attack	Nausea
Anxiety	Brain Fog	Hearing Loss	Hyperacusis
Fatigue	Balance	Co-ordination	Stress
Headache	Migraine	Nystagmus	Disequilibrium
Ear Fullness/ Pressure/Pain	Vision Difficulties	Physical Impairment	Vestibular Migraine
Vomiting	Depression	BPPV*	Diarrhea
PPPD*	Jaw Click/Pain	Neck Pain	Motion Sensitivity
Sweating	Speech Difficulty	Monthly Cycle	

What time did your symptoms start? ____________

Tinnitus: L R How many noises? ______ Loudness Scale: 1 2 3 4 5

Possible Meniere's Symptom Triggers Today:

Physical: ____________

____

____

____________ Pollen, Mold, Dust, Trees, Grass, Ragweed

Visual: ____________

____

____

Emotional: ____________

____

____

What Helped Me?

Medication/s & Time Taken		Other	
		Prayer	Rest
		Meditation	Friend/s
		Self-care	Family
		Exercise	Pet/s
		Mindfulness	Vestibular Rehab
		Gratitude	Hearing Device

Duration of Vertigo ______ minutes ______ hours ______ days

Severity of Vertigo 1 2 3 4 5 - I HATE you, vertigo!

New Symptoms? ____________

____

What I Accomplished Today – Something to Celebrate! ♡

____

____

____

Three Things I am Thankful for Today:

1.
2.
3.

MONTH: January February March April May June July August September October November December

Day: Monday Tuesday Wednesday Thursday Friday Saturday Sunday

Date: ______ **Season:** Summer Autumn/Fall Winter Spring

Temperature: Low ________ High ________

Barometer: 9am__________ 9pm__________ **Humidity** ______________

Sunny	Cloudy	Rain	Showers	Windy
Snow	Storm	Humid	Dry	

Food & Fluid Intake (be mindful of salt):

Breakfast			
Lunch			
Dinner			
Fluid Intake	Water - ______		
Snacks			

Symptoms:

Tinnitus	Vertigo	Drop Attack	Nausea
Anxiety	Brain Fog	Hearing Loss	Hyperacusis
Fatigue	Balance	Co-ordination	Stress
Headache	Migraine	Nystagmus	Disequilibrium
Ear Fullness/ Pressure/Pain	Vision Difficulties	Physical Impairment	Vestibular Migraine
Vomiting	Depression	BPPV*	Diarrhea
PPPD*	Jaw Click/Pain	Neck Pain	Motion Sensitivity
Sweating	Speech Difficulty	Monthly Cycle	

What time did your symptoms start? ____________________

Tinnitus: L R How many noises? ______ Loudness Scale: 1 2 3 4 5

Possible Meniere's Symptom Triggers Today:

Physical: ____________________

____

____

____________________ Pollen, Mold, Dust, Trees, Grass, Ragweed

Visual: ____________________

____

____

Emotional: ____________________

____

____

What Helped Me?

Medication/s & Time Taken		Other	
		Prayer	Rest
		Meditation	Friend/s
		Self-care	Family
		Exercise	Pet/s
		Mindfulness	Vestibular Rehab
		Gratitude	Hearing Device

Duration of Vertigo ______ minutes ______ hours______ days

Severity of Vertigo 1 2 3 4 5 - I HATE you, vertigo!

New Symptoms? ____________________

____

What I Accomplished Today - Something to Celebrate! ♡

____

____

____

Three Things I am Thankful for Today:

1.
2.
3.

MONTH: January February March April May June July August September October November December

Day: Monday Tuesday Wednesday Thursday Friday Saturday Sunday
Date: ______ **Season:** Summer Autumn/Fall Winter Spring
Temperature: Low _______ High _______
Barometer: 9am__________ 9pm__________ **Humidity** ___________

Sunny	Cloudy	Rain	Showers	Windy
Snow	Storm	Humid	Dry	

Food & Fluid Intake (be mindful of salt):

Breakfast			
Lunch			
Dinner			
Fluid Intake	Water - _____		
Snacks			

Symptoms:

Tinnitus	Vertigo	Drop Attack	Nausea
Anxiety	Brain Fog	Hearing Loss	Hyperacusis
Fatigue	Balance	Co-ordination	Stress
Headache	Migraine	Nystagmus	Disequilibrium
Ear Fullness/ Pressure/Pain	Vision Difficulties	Physical Impairment	Vestibular Migraine
Vomiting	Depression	BPPV*	Diarrhea
PPPD*	Jaw Click/Pain	Neck Pain	Motion Sensitivity
Sweating	Speech Difficulty	Monthly Cycle	

What time did your symptoms start? ____________

Tinnitus: L R How many noises? ______ Loudness Scale: 1 2 3 4 5

Possible Meniere's Symptom Triggers Today:

Physical: ____________

____

____

____________ Pollen, Mold, Dust, Trees, Grass, Ragweed

Visual: ____________

____

____

Emotional: ____________

____

____

What Helped Me?

Medication/s & Time Taken		Other	
		Prayer	Rest
		Meditation	Friend/s
		Self-care	Family
		Exercise	Pet/s
		Mindfulness	Vestibular Rehab
		Gratitude	Hearing Device

Duration of Vertigo ______ minutes ______ hours______ days

Severity of Vertigo 1 2 3 4 5 - I HATE you, vertigo!

New Symptoms? ____________

____

What I Accomplished Today – Something to Celebrate! ♡

____

____

____

Three Things I am Thankful for Today:

1.
2.
3.

MONTH: January February March April May June July August September October November December

Day: Monday Tuesday Wednesday Thursday Friday Saturday Sunday
Date: _______ **Season:** Summer Autumn/Fall Winter Spring
Temperature: Low _______ High _______
Barometer: 9am__________ 9pm__________ **Humidity** ___________

Sunny	Cloudy	Rain	Showers	Windy
Snow	Storm	Humid	Dry	

Food & Fluid Intake (be mindful of salt):

Breakfast			
Lunch			
Dinner			
Fluid Intake	Water - ______		
Snacks			

Symptoms:

Tinnitus	Vertigo	Drop Attack	Nausea
Anxiety	Brain Fog	Hearing Loss	Hyperacusis
Fatigue	Balance	Co-ordination	Stress
Headache	Migraine	Nystagmus	Disequilibrium
Ear Fullness/ Pressure/Pain	Vision Difficulties	Physical Impairment	Vestibular Migraine
Vomiting	Depression	BPPV*	Diarrhea
PPPD*	Jaw Click/Pain	Neck Pain	Motion Sensitivity
Sweating	Speech Difficulty	Monthly Cycle	

What time did your symptoms start? ____________

Tinnitus: L R How many noises? _______ Loudness Scale: 1 2 3 4 5

Possible Meniere's Symptom Triggers Today:

Physical: ____________

____

____

____________ Pollen, Mold, Dust, Trees, Grass, Ragweed

Visual: ____________

____

____

Emotional: ____________

____

____

What Helped Me?

Medication/s & Time Taken		Other	
		Prayer	Rest
		Meditation	Friend/s
		Self-care	Family
		Exercise	Pet/s
		Mindfulness	Vestibular Rehab
		Gratitude	Hearing Device

Duration of Vertigo ______ minutes ______ hours______ days

Severity of Vertigo 1 2 3 4 5 - I HATE you, vertigo!

New Symptoms? ____________

____

What I Accomplished Today - Something to Celebrate! ♡

____

____

____

Three Things I am Thankful for Today:

1.
2.
3.

MONTH: January February March April May June July August September October November December

Day: Monday Tuesday Wednesday Thursday Friday Saturday Sunday
Date: ______ **Season:** Summer Autumn/Fall Winter Spring
Temperature: Low ________ High ________
Barometer: 9am__________ 9pm_________ **Humidity** ____________

Sunny	Cloudy	Rain	Showers	Windy
Snow	Storm	Humid	Dry	

Food & Fluid Intake (be mindful of salt):

Breakfast			
Lunch			
Dinner			
Fluid Intake	Water - ________		
Snacks			

Symptoms:

Tinnitus	Vertigo	Drop Attack	Nausea
Anxiety	Brain Fog	Hearing Loss	Hyperacusis
Fatigue	Balance	Co-ordination	Stress
Headache	Migraine	Nystagmus	Disequilibrium
Ear Fullness/ Pressure/Pain	Vision Difficulties	Physical Impairment	Vestibular Migraine
Vomiting	Depression	BPPV*	Diarrhea
PPPD*	Jaw Click/Pain	Neck Pain	Motion Sensitivity
Sweating	Speech Difficulty	Monthly Cycle	

What time did your symptoms start? ____________

Tinnitus: L R How many noises? ______ Loudness Scale: 1 2 3 4 5

Possible Meniere's Symptom Triggers Today:

Physical: ____________

____

____

____________ Pollen, Mold, Dust, Trees, Grass, Ragweed

Visual: ____________

____

____

Emotional: ____________

____

____

What Helped Me?

Medication/s & Time Taken		Other	
		Prayer	Rest
		Meditation	Friend/s
		Self-care	Family
		Exercise	Pet/s
		Mindfulness	Vestibular Rehab
		Gratitude	Hearing Device

Duration of Vertigo ______ minutes ______ hours ______ days

Severity of Vertigo 1 2 3 4 5 - I HATE you, vertigo!

New Symptoms? ____________

____

What I Accomplished Today - Something to Celebrate! ♡

____

____

____

Three Things I am Thankful for Today:

1.
2.
3.

MONTH: January February March April May June July August September October November December

Day: Monday Tuesday Wednesday Thursday Friday Saturday Sunday
Date: ______ **Season:** Summer Autumn/Fall Winter Spring
Temperature: Low _______ High _______
Barometer: 9am__________ 9pm__________ **Humidity** ___________

Sunny	Cloudy	Rain	Showers	Windy
Snow	Storm	Humid	Dry	

Food & Fluid Intake (be mindful of salt):

Breakfast			
Lunch			
Dinner			
Fluid Intake	Water - ____		
Snacks			

Symptoms:

Tinnitus	Vertigo	Drop Attack	Nausea
Anxiety	Brain Fog	Hearing Loss	Hyperacusis
Fatigue	Balance	Co-ordination	Stress
Headache	Migraine	Nystagmus	Disequilibrium
Ear Fullness/ Pressure/Pain	Vision Difficulties	Physical Impairment	Vestibular Migraine
Vomiting	Depression	BPPV*	Diarrhea
PPPD*	Jaw Click/Pain	Neck Pain	Motion Sensitivity
Sweating	Speech Difficulty	Monthly Cycle	

What time did your symptoms start? ______

Tinnitus: L R How many noises? ______ Loudness Scale: 1 2 3 4 5

Possible Meniere's Symptom Triggers Today:

Physical: ______

______ Pollen, Mold, Dust, Trees, Grass, Ragweed

Visual: ______

Emotional: ______

What Helped Me?

Medication/s & Time Taken		Other	
		Prayer	Rest
		Meditation	Friend/s
		Self-care	Family
		Exercise	Pet/s
		Mindfulness	Vestibular Rehab
		Gratitude	Hearing Device

Duration of Vertigo ______ minutes ______ hours ______ days

Severity of Vertigo 1 2 3 4 5 - I HATE you, vertigo!

New Symptoms? ______

What I Accomplished Today - Something to Celebrate! ♡

______

Three Things I am Thankful for Today:

1.
2.
3.

MONTH: January February March April May June July August September October November December

Day: Monday Tuesday Wednesday Thursday Friday Saturday Sunday
Date: _______ **Season:** Summer Autumn/Fall Winter Spring
Temperature: Low _______ High _______
Barometer: 9am_______ 9pm_______ **Humidity** _____________

Sunny	Cloudy	Rain	Showers	Windy
Snow	Storm	Humid	Dry	

Food & Fluid Intake (be mindful of salt):

Breakfast			
Lunch			
Dinner			
Fluid Intake	Water - _______		
Snacks			

Symptoms:

Tinnitus	Vertigo	Drop Attack	Nausea
Anxiety	Brain Fog	Hearing Loss	Hyperacusis
Fatigue	Balance	Co-ordination	Stress
Headache	Migraine	Nystagmus	Disequilibrium
Ear Fullness/ Pressure/Pain	Vision Difficulties	Physical Impairment	Vestibular Migraine
Vomiting	Depression	BPPV*	Diarrhea
PPPD*	Jaw Click/Pain	Neck Pain	Motion Sensitivity
Sweating	Speech Difficulty	Monthly Cycle	

What time did your symptoms start? ____________

Tinnitus: L R How many noises? ________ Loudness Scale: 1 2 3 4 5

Possible Meniere's Symptom Triggers Today:

Physical: ____________

____

____

____________ Pollen, Mold, Dust, Trees, Grass, Ragweed

Visual: ____________

____

____

Emotional: ____________

____

____

What Helped Me?

Medication/s & Time Taken		Other	
		Prayer	Rest
		Meditation	Friend/s
		Self-care	Family
		Exercise	Pet/s
		Mindfulness	Vestibular Rehab
		Gratitude	Hearing Device

Duration of Vertigo ______ minutes ______ hours______ days

Severity of Vertigo 1 2 3 4 5 - I HATE you, vertigo!

New Symptoms? ____________

____

What I Accomplished Today – Something to Celebrate! ♡

____

____

____

Three Things I am Thankful for Today:

1.
2.
3.

MONTH: January February March April May June July August September October November December

Day: Monday Tuesday Wednesday Thursday Friday Saturday Sunday

Date: ______ **Season:** Summer Autumn/Fall Winter Spring

Temperature: Low _______ High _______

Barometer: 9am__________ 9pm_________ **Humidity** ____________

Sunny	Cloudy	Rain	Showers	Windy
Snow	Storm	Humid	Dry	

Food & Fluid Intake (be mindful of salt):

Breakfast			
Lunch			
Dinner			
Fluid Intake	Water - _______		
Snacks			

Symptoms:

Tinnitus	Vertigo	Drop Attack	Nausea
Anxiety	Brain Fog	Hearing Loss	Hyperacusis
Fatigue	Balance	Co-ordination	Stress
Headache	Migraine	Nystagmus	Disequilibrium
Ear Fullness/ Pressure/Pain	Vision Difficulties	Physical Impairment	Vestibular Migraine
Vomiting	Depression	BPPV*	Diarrhea
PPPD*	Jaw Click/Pain	Neck Pain	Motion Sensitivity
Sweating	Speech Difficulty	Monthly Cycle	

What time did your symptoms start? ____________________

Tinnitus: L R How many noises? _______ Loudness Scale: 1 2 3 4 5

Possible Meniere's Symptom Triggers Today:

Physical: ____________________

____

____

____________________ Pollen, Mold, Dust, Trees, Grass, Ragweed

Visual: ____________________

____

____

Emotional: ____________________

____

____

What Helped Me?

Medication/s & Time Taken		Other	
		Prayer	Rest
		Meditation	Friend/s
		Self-care	Family
		Exercise	Pet/s
		Mindfulness	Vestibular Rehab
		Gratitude	Hearing Device

Duration of Vertigo ______ minutes ______ hours ______ days

Severity of Vertigo 1 2 3 4 5 - I HATE you, vertigo!

New Symptoms? ____________________

____

What I Accomplished Today – Something to Celebrate! ♡

____

____

____

Three Things I am Thankful for Today:

1.
2.
3.

MONTH: January February March April May June July August September October November December

Day: Monday Tuesday Wednesday Thursday Friday Saturday Sunday
Date: ______ **Season:** Summer Autumn/Fall Winter Spring
Temperature: Low _______ High _______
Barometer: 9am_______ 9pm_______ **Humidity** ___________

Sunny	Cloudy	Rain	Showers	Windy
Snow	Storm	Humid	Dry	

Food & Fluid Intake (be mindful of salt):

Breakfast			
Lunch			
Dinner			
Fluid Intake	Water - ____		
Snacks			

Symptoms:

Tinnitus	Vertigo	Drop Attack	Nausea
Anxiety	Brain Fog	Hearing Loss	Hyperacusis
Fatigue	Balance	Co-ordination	Stress
Headache	Migraine	Nystagmus	Disequilibrium
Ear Fullness/ Pressure/Pain	Vision Difficulties	Physical Impairment	Vestibular Migraine
Vomiting	Depression	BPPV*	Diarrhea
PPPD*	Jaw Click/Pain	Neck Pain	Motion Sensitivity
Sweating	Speech Difficulty	Monthly Cycle	

What time did your symptoms start? ____________________

Tinnitus: L R How many noises? ______ Loudness Scale: 1 2 3 4 5

Possible Meniere's Symptom Triggers Today:

Physical: ____________________

____

____

____________________ Pollen, Mold, Dust, Trees, Grass, Ragweed

Visual: ____________________

____

Emotional: ____________________

____

____

What Helped Me?

Medication/s & Time Taken		Other	
		Prayer	Rest
		Meditation	Friend/s
		Self-care	Family
		Exercise	Pet/s
		Mindfulness	Vestibular Rehab
		Gratitude	Hearing Device

Duration of Vertigo ______ minutes ______ hours ______ days

Severity of Vertigo 1 2 3 4 5 - I HATE you, vertigo!

New Symptoms? ____________________

What I Accomplished Today - Something to Celebrate! ♡

____

____

____

Three Things I am Thankful for Today:

1.
2.
3.

MONTH: January February March April May June July August September October November December

Day: Monday Tuesday Wednesday Thursday Friday Saturday Sunday
Date: ______ **Season:** Summer Autumn/Fall Winter Spring
Temperature: Low _______ High _______
Barometer: 9am_________ 9pm_________ **Humidity**___________

Sunny	Cloudy	Rain	Showers	Windy
Snow	Storm	Humid	Dry	

Food & Fluid Intake (be mindful of salt):

Breakfast			
Lunch			
Dinner			
Fluid Intake	Water - ______		
Snacks			

Symptoms:

Tinnitus	Vertigo	Drop Attack	Nausea
Anxiety	Brain Fog	Hearing Loss	Hyperacusis
Fatigue	Balance	Co-ordination	Stress
Headache	Migraine	Nystagmus	Disequilibrium
Ear Fullness/ Pressure/Pain	Vision Difficulties	Physical Impairment	Vestibular Migraine
Vomiting	Depression	BPPV*	Diarrhea
PPPD*	Jaw Click/Pain	Neck Pain	Motion Sensitivity
Sweating	Speech Difficulty	Monthly Cycle	

What time did your symptoms start? ____________________

Tinnitus: L R How many noises? _______ Loudness Scale: 1 2 3 4 5

Possible Meniere's Symptom Triggers Today:

Physical: ____________________

____

____

____________________ Pollen, Mold, Dust, Trees, Grass, Ragweed

Visual: ____________________

____

____

Emotional: ____________________

____

____

What Helped Me?

Medication/s & Time Taken		Other	
		Prayer	Rest
		Meditation	Friend/s
		Self-care	Family
		Exercise	Pet/s
		Mindfulness	Vestibular Rehab
		Gratitude	Hearing Device

Duration of Vertigo ______ minutes ______ hours ______ days

Severity of Vertigo 1 2 3 4 5 - I HATE you, vertigo!

New Symptoms? ____________________

____

What I Accomplished Today – Something to Celebrate! ♡

____

____

____

Three Things I am Thankful for Today:

1.
2.
3.

MONTH: January February March April May June July August September October November December

Day: Monday Tuesday Wednesday Thursday Friday Saturday Sunday
Date: ______ **Season:** Summer Autumn/Fall Winter Spring
Temperature: Low _______ High _______
Barometer: 9am_________ 9pm________ **Humidity** ____________

Sunny	Cloudy	Rain	Showers	Windy
Snow	Storm	Humid	Dry	

Food & Fluid Intake (be mindful of salt):

Breakfast			
Lunch			
Dinner			
Fluid Intake	Water - ______		
Snacks			

Symptoms:

Tinnitus	Vertigo	Drop Attack	Nausea
Anxiety	Brain Fog	Hearing Loss	Hyperacusis
Fatigue	Balance	Co-ordination	Stress
Headache	Migraine	Nystagmus	Disequilibrium
Ear Fullness/ Pressure/Pain	Vision Difficulties	Physical Impairment	Vestibular Migraine
Vomiting	Depression	BPPV*	Diarrhea
PPPD*	Jaw Click/Pain	Neck Pain	Motion Sensitivity
Sweating	Speech Difficulty	Monthly Cycle	

What time did your symptoms start? ______________

Tinnitus: L R How many noises? ______ Loudness Scale: 1 2 3 4 5

Possible Meniere's Symptom Triggers Today:

Physical: ______________________________

______________________________ Pollen, Mold, Dust, Trees, Grass, Ragweed

Visual: ______________________________

Emotional: ______________________________

What Helped Me?

Medication/s & Time Taken		Other	
		Prayer	Rest
		Meditation	Friend/s
		Self-care	Family
		Exercise	Pet/s
		Mindfulness	Vestibular Rehab
		Gratitude	Hearing Device

Duration of Vertigo ______ minutes ______ hours ______ days

Severity of Vertigo 1 2 3 4 5 - I HATE you, vertigo!

New Symptoms? ______________________________

What I Accomplished Today - Something to Celebrate! ♡

Three Things I am Thankful for Today:

1.
2.
3.

MONTH: January February March April May June July August September October November December

Day: Monday Tuesday Wednesday Thursday Friday Saturday Sunday
Date: _______ **Season:** Summer Autumn/Fall Winter Spring
Temperature: Low ________ High ________
Barometer: 9am________ 9pm________ **Humidity** ____________

Sunny	Cloudy	Rain	Showers	Windy
Snow	Storm	Humid	Dry	

Food & Fluid Intake (be mindful of salt):

Breakfast			
Lunch			
Dinner			
Fluid Intake	Water - ______		
Snacks			

Symptoms:

Tinnitus	Vertigo	Drop Attack	Nausea
Anxiety	Brain Fog	Hearing Loss	Hyperacusis
Fatigue	Balance	Co-ordination	Stress
Headache	Migraine	Nystagmus	Disequilibrium
Ear Fullness/ Pressure/Pain	Vision Difficulties	Physical Impairment	Vestibular Migraine
Vomiting	Depression	BPPV*	Diarrhea
PPPD*	Jaw Click/Pain	Neck Pain	Motion Sensitivity
Sweating	Speech Difficulty	Monthly Cycle	

What time did your symptoms start? ______________________

Tinnitus: L R How many noises? ________ Loudness Scale: 1 2 3 4 5

Possible Meniere's Symptom Triggers Today:

Physical: ______________________

____

____

______________________ Pollen, Mold, Dust, Trees, Grass, Ragweed

Visual: ______________________

____

____

Emotional: ______________________

____

____

What Helped Me?

Medication/s & Time Taken		Other	
		Prayer	Rest
		Meditation	Friend/s
		Self-care	Family
		Exercise	Pet/s
		Mindfulness	Vestibular Rehab
		Gratitude	Hearing Device

Duration of Vertigo ______ minutes ______ hours______ days

Severity of Vertigo 1 2 3 4 5 - I HATE you, vertigo!

New Symptoms? ______________________

____

What I Accomplished Today – Something to Celebrate! ♡

____

____

____

Three Things I am Thankful for Today:

1.
2.
3.

MONTH: January February March April May June July August September October November December

Day: Monday Tuesday Wednesday Thursday Friday Saturday Sunday
Date: ______ **Season:** Summer Autumn/Fall Winter Spring
Temperature: Low ______ High ______
Barometer: 9am______ 9pm______ **Humidity** ______

Sunny	Cloudy	Rain	Showers	Windy
Snow	Storm	Humid	Dry	

Food & Fluid Intake (be mindful of salt):

Breakfast			
Lunch			
Dinner			
Fluid Intake	Water - ______		
Snacks			

Symptoms:

Tinnitus	Vertigo	Drop Attack	Nausea
Anxiety	Brain Fog	Hearing Loss	Hyperacusis
Fatigue	Balance	Co-ordination	Stress
Headache	Migraine	Nystagmus	Disequilibrium
Ear Fullness/ Pressure/Pain	Vision Difficulties	Physical Impairment	Vestibular Migraine
Vomiting	Depression	BPPV*	Diarrhea
PPPD*	Jaw Click/Pain	Neck Pain	Motion Sensitivity
Sweating	Speech Difficulty	Monthly Cycle	

What time did your symptoms start? ______________________

Tinnitus: L R How many noises? _______ Loudness Scale: 1 2 3 4 5

Possible Meniere's Symptom Triggers Today:

Physical: ____

____

____

__________________________ Pollen, Mold, Dust, Trees, Grass, Ragweed

Visual: ____

____

____

Emotional: ____

____

____

What Helped Me?

Medication/s & Time Taken		Other	
		Prayer	Rest
		Meditation	Friend/s
		Self-care	Family
		Exercise	Pet/s
		Mindfulness	Vestibular Rehab
		Gratitude	Hearing Device

Duration of Vertigo ______ minutes ______ hours______ days

Severity of Vertigo 1 2 3 4 5 - I HATE you, vertigo!

New Symptoms? ____

____

What I Accomplished Today – Something to Celebrate! ♡

____

____

____

Three Things I am Thankful for Today:

1.
2.
3.

MONTH: January February March April May June July August September October November December

Day: Monday Tuesday Wednesday Thursday Friday Saturday Sunday
Date: ______ **Season:** Summer Autumn/Fall Winter Spring
Temperature: Low _______ High _______
Barometer: 9am_________ 9pm_________ **Humidity** ____________

Sunny	Cloudy	Rain	Showers	Windy
Snow	Storm	Humid	Dry	

Food & Fluid Intake (be mindful of salt):

Breakfast			
Lunch			
Dinner			
Fluid Intake	Water - ______		
Snacks			

Symptoms:

Tinnitus	Vertigo	Drop Attack	Nausea
Anxiety	Brain Fog	Hearing Loss	Hyperacusis
Fatigue	Balance	Co-ordination	Stress
Headache	Migraine	Nystagmus	Disequilibrium
Ear Fullness/ Pressure/Pain	Vision Difficulties	Physical Impairment	Vestibular Migraine
Vomiting	Depression	BPPV*	Diarrhea
PPPD*	Jaw Click/Pain	Neck Pain	Motion Sensitivity
Sweating	Speech Difficulty	Monthly Cycle	

What time did your symptoms start? ________________________

Tinnitus: L R How many noises? ______ Loudness Scale: 1 2 3 4 5

Possible Meniere's Symptom Triggers Today:

Physical: ____

____

____

________________________ Pollen, Mold, Dust, Trees, Grass, Ragweed

Visual: ____

____

Emotional: ____

____

____

What Helped Me?

Medication/s & Time Taken		Other	
		Prayer	Rest
		Meditation	Friend/s
		Self-care	Family
		Exercise	Pet/s
		Mindfulness	Vestibular Rehab
		Gratitude	Hearing Device

Duration of Vertigo ______ minutes ______ hours ______ days

Severity of Vertigo 1 2 3 4 5 - I HATE you, vertigo!

New Symptoms? ____

____

What I Accomplished Today - Something to Celebrate! ♡

____

____

____

Three Things I am Thankful for Today:

1.
2.
3.

MONTH: January February March April May June July August September October November December

Day: Monday Tuesday Wednesday Thursday Friday Saturday Sunday
Date: ______ **Season:** Summer Autumn/Fall Winter Spring
Temperature: Low _______ High _______
Barometer: 9am_______ 9pm_______ **Humidity** ___________

Sunny	Cloudy	Rain	Showers	Windy
Snow	Storm	Humid	Dry	

Food & Fluid Intake (be mindful of salt):

Breakfast			
Lunch			
Dinner			
Fluid Intake	Water - ______		
Snacks			

Symptoms:

Tinnitus	Vertigo	Drop Attack	Nausea
Anxiety	Brain Fog	Hearing Loss	Hyperacusis
Fatigue	Balance	Co-ordination	Stress
Headache	Migraine	Nystagmus	Disequilibrium
Ear Fullness/ Pressure/Pain	Vision Difficulties	Physical Impairment	Vestibular Migraine
Vomiting	Depression	BPPV*	Diarrhea
PPPD*	Jaw Click/Pain	Neck Pain	Motion Sensitivity
Sweating	Speech Difficulty	Monthly Cycle	

What time did your symptoms start? ______________________

Tinnitus: L R How many noises? ______ Loudness Scale: 1 2 3 4 5

Possible Meniere's Symptom Triggers Today:

Physical: ______________________

____

____

______________________ Pollen, Mold, Dust, Trees, Grass, Ragweed

Visual: ______________________

____

____

Emotional: ______________________

____

____

What Helped Me?

Medication/s & Time Taken		Other	
		Prayer	Rest
		Meditation	Friend/s
		Self-care	Family
		Exercise	Pet/s
		Mindfulness	Vestibular Rehab
		Gratitude	Hearing Device

Duration of Vertigo ______ minutes ______ hours ______ days

Severity of Vertigo 1 2 3 4 5 - I HATE you, vertigo!

New Symptoms? ______________________

____

What I Accomplished Today - Something to Celebrate! ♡

____

____

____

Three Things I am Thankful for Today:

1.
2.
3.

MONTH: January February March April May June July August September October November December

Day: Monday Tuesday Wednesday Thursday Friday Saturday Sunday
Date: ______ **Season:** Summer Autumn/Fall Winter Spring
Temperature: Low _______ High _______
Barometer: 9am_________ 9pm_________ **Humidity** ____________

Sunny	Cloudy	Rain	Showers	Windy
Snow	Storm	Humid	Dry	

Food & Fluid Intake (be mindful of salt):

Breakfast			
Lunch			
Dinner			
Fluid Intake	Water - _____		
Snacks			

Symptoms:

Tinnitus	Vertigo	Drop Attack	Nausea
Anxiety	Brain Fog	Hearing Loss	Hyperacusis
Fatigue	Balance	Co-ordination	Stress
Headache	Migraine	Nystagmus	Disequilibrium
Ear Fullness/ Pressure/Pain	Vision Difficulties	Physical Impairment	Vestibular Migraine
Vomiting	Depression	BPPV*	Diarrhea
PPPD*	Jaw Click/Pain	Neck Pain	Motion Sensitivity
Sweating	Speech Difficulty	Monthly Cycle	

What time did your symptoms start? ______________

Tinnitus: L R How many noises? _______ Loudness Scale: 1 2 3 4 5

Possible Meniere's Symptom Triggers Today:

Physical: ____

____

____

______________________ Pollen, Mold, Dust, Trees, Grass, Ragweed

Visual: ____

____

____

Emotional: ____

____

____

What Helped Me?

Medication/s & Time Taken		Other	
		Prayer	Rest
		Meditation	Friend/s
		Self-care	Family
		Exercise	Pet/s
		Mindfulness	Vestibular Rehab
		Gratitude	Hearing Device

Duration of Vertigo ______ minutes ______ hours______ days

Severity of Vertigo 1 2 3 4 5 - I HATE you, vertigo!

New Symptoms? ______________________________

____

What I Accomplished Today - Something to Celebrate! ♡

____

____

____

Three Things I am Thankful for Today:

1.
2.
3.

MONTH: January February March April May June July August September October November December

Day: Monday Tuesday Wednesday Thursday Friday Saturday Sunday
Date: ______ **Season:** Summer Autumn/Fall Winter Spring
Temperature: Low ________ High ________
Barometer: 9am__________ 9pm_________ **Humidity** ______________

Sunny	Cloudy	Rain	Showers	Windy
Snow	Storm	Humid	Dry	

Food & Fluid Intake (be mindful of salt):

Breakfast			
Lunch			
Dinner			
Fluid Intake	Water - _______		
Snacks			

Symptoms:

Tinnitus	Vertigo	Drop Attack	Nausea
Anxiety	Brain Fog	Hearing Loss	Hyperacusis
Fatigue	Balance	Co-ordination	Stress
Headache	Migraine	Nystagmus	Disequilibrium
Ear Fullness/ Pressure/Pain	Vision Difficulties	Physical Impairment	Vestibular Migraine
Vomiting	Depression	BPPV*	Diarrhea
PPPD*	Jaw Click/Pain	Neck Pain	Motion Sensitivity
Sweating	Speech Difficulty	Monthly Cycle	

What time did your symptoms start? ___________________

Tinnitus: L R How many noises? _______ Loudness Scale: 1 2 3 4 5

Possible Meniere's Symptom Triggers Today:

Physical: ____

____

____

___________________________ Pollen, Mold, Dust, Trees, Grass, Ragweed

Visual: ____

____

Emotional: ____

____

____

What Helped Me?

Medication/s & Time Taken		Other	
		Prayer	Rest
		Meditation	Friend/s
		Self-care	Family
		Exercise	Pet/s
		Mindfulness	Vestibular Rehab
		Gratitude	Hearing Device

Duration of Vertigo _______ minutes _______ hours_______ days

Severity of Vertigo 1 2 3 4 5 - I HATE you, vertigo!

New Symptoms? ____

____

What I Accomplished Today - Something to Celebrate! ♡

____

____

____

Three Things I am Thankful for Today:

1.
2.
3.

MONTH: January February March April May June July August September October November December

Day: Monday Tuesday Wednesday Thursday Friday Saturday Sunday

Date: ______ **Season:** Summer Autumn/Fall Winter Spring

Temperature: Low ______ High ______

Barometer: 9am______ 9pm______ **Humidity** ______

Sunny	Cloudy	Rain	Showers	Windy
Snow	Storm	Humid	Dry	

Food & Fluid Intake (be mindful of salt):

Breakfast			
Lunch			
Dinner			
Fluid Intake	Water - ______		
Snacks			

Symptoms:

Tinnitus	Vertigo	Drop Attack	Nausea
Anxiety	Brain Fog	Hearing Loss	Hyperacusis
Fatigue	Balance	Co-ordination	Stress
Headache	Migraine	Nystagmus	Disequilibrium
Ear Fullness/ Pressure/Pain	Vision Difficulties	Physical Impairment	Vestibular Migraine
Vomiting	Depression	BPPV*	Diarrhea
PPPD*	Jaw Click/Pain	Neck Pain	Motion Sensitivity
Sweating	Speech Difficulty	Monthly Cycle	

What time did your symptoms start? ____________

Tinnitus: L R How many noises? ______ Loudness Scale: 1 2 3 4 5

Possible Meniere's Symptom Triggers Today:

Physical: ____________

____

____

____________ Pollen, Mold, Dust, Trees, Grass, Ragweed

Visual: ____________

____

____

Emotional: ____________

____

____

What Helped Me?

Medication/s & Time Taken		Other	
		Prayer	Rest
		Meditation	Friend/s
		Self-care	Family
		Exercise	Pet/s
		Mindfulness	Vestibular Rehab
		Gratitude	Hearing Device

Duration of Vertigo ______ minutes ______ hours ______ days

Severity of Vertigo 1 2 3 4 5 - I HATE you, vertigo!

New Symptoms? ____________

____

What I Accomplished Today - Something to Celebrate! ♡

____

____

____

Three Things I am Thankful for Today:

1.
2.
3.

MONTH: January February March April May June July August September October November December

Day: Monday Tuesday Wednesday Thursday Friday Saturday Sunday
Date: ______ **Season:** Summer Autumn/Fall Winter Spring
Temperature: Low ______ High ______
Barometer: 9am ______ 9pm ______ **Humidity** ______

Sunny	Cloudy	Rain	Showers	Windy
Snow	Storm	Humid	Dry	

Food & Fluid Intake (be mindful of salt):

Breakfast			
Lunch			
Dinner			
Fluid Intake	Water - ______		
Snacks			

Symptoms:

Tinnitus	Vertigo	Drop Attack	Nausea
Anxiety	Brain Fog	Hearing Loss	Hyperacusis
Fatigue	Balance	Co-ordination	Stress
Headache	Migraine	Nystagmus	Disequilibrium
Ear Fullness/ Pressure/Pain	Vision Difficulties	Physical Impairment	Vestibular Migraine
Vomiting	Depression	BPPV*	Diarrhea
PPPD*	Jaw Click/Pain	Neck Pain	Motion Sensitivity
Sweating	Speech Difficulty	Monthly Cycle	

What time did your symptoms start? ______________________

Tinnitus: L R How many noises? ______ Loudness Scale: 1 2 3 4 5

Possible Meniere's Symptom Triggers Today:

Physical: ______________________

____

____

______________________ Pollen, Mold, Dust, Trees, Grass, Ragweed

Visual: ______________________

____

____

Emotional: ______________________

____

____

What Helped Me?

Medication/s & Time Taken		Other	
		Prayer	Rest
		Meditation	Friend/s
		Self-care	Family
		Exercise	Pet/s
		Mindfulness	Vestibular Rehab
		Gratitude	Hearing Device

Duration of Vertigo ______ minutes ______ hours______ days

Severity of Vertigo 1 2 3 4 5 - I HATE you, vertigo!

New Symptoms? ______________________

____

What I Accomplished Today – Something to Celebrate! ♡

____

____

____

Three Things I am Thankful for Today:

1.
2.
3.

MONTH: January February March April May June July August September October November December

Day: Monday Tuesday Wednesday Thursday Friday Saturday Sunday
Date: ______ **Season:** Summer Autumn/Fall Winter Spring
Temperature: Low _______ High _______
Barometer: 9am_________ 9pm________ **Humidity** ____________

Sunny	Cloudy	Rain	Showers	Windy
Snow	Storm	Humid	Dry	

Food & Fluid Intake (be mindful of salt):

Breakfast			
Lunch			
Dinner			
Fluid Intake	Water - _____		
Snacks			

Symptoms:

Tinnitus	Vertigo	Drop Attack	Nausea
Anxiety	Brain Fog	Hearing Loss	Hyperacusis
Fatigue	Balance	Co-ordination	Stress
Headache	Migraine	Nystagmus	Disequilibrium
Ear Fullness/ Pressure/Pain	Vision Difficulties	Physical Impairment	Vestibular Migraine
Vomiting	Depression	BPPV*	Diarrhea
PPPD*	Jaw Click/Pain	Neck Pain	Motion Sensitivity
Sweating	Speech Difficulty	Monthly Cycle	

What time did your symptoms start? ____________________

Tinnitus: L R How many noises? ______ Loudness Scale: 1 2 3 4 5

Possible Meniere's Symptom Triggers Today:

Physical: ____________________

____

____

____________________ Pollen, Mold, Dust, Trees, Grass, Ragweed

Visual: ____________________

____

____

Emotional: ____________________

____

____

What Helped Me?

Medication/s & Time Taken		Other	
		Prayer	Rest
		Meditation	Friend/s
		Self-care	Family
		Exercise	Pet/s
		Mindfulness	Vestibular Rehab
		Gratitude	Hearing Device

Duration of Vertigo ______ minutes ______ hours______ days

Severity of Vertigo 1 2 3 4 5 - I HATE you, vertigo!

New Symptoms? ____________________

____

What I Accomplished Today - Something to Celebrate! ♡

____

____

____

Three Things I am Thankful for Today:

1.
2.
3.

MONTH: January February March April May June July August September October November December

Day: Monday Tuesday Wednesday Thursday Friday Saturday Sunday

Date: ______ **Season:** Summer Autumn/Fall Winter Spring

Temperature: Low ________ High ________

Barometer: 9am__________ 9pm__________ **Humidity** ____________

Sunny	Cloudy	Rain	Showers	Windy
Snow	Storm	Humid	Dry	

Food & Fluid Intake (be mindful of salt):

Breakfast			
Lunch			
Dinner			
Fluid Intake	Water - ______		
Snacks			

Symptoms:

Tinnitus	Vertigo	Drop Attack	Nausea
Anxiety	Brain Fog	Hearing Loss	Hyperacusis
Fatigue	Balance	Co-ordination	Stress
Headache	Migraine	Nystagmus	Disequilibrium
Ear Fullness/ Pressure/Pain	Vision Difficulties	Physical Impairment	Vestibular Migraine
Vomiting	Depression	BPPV*	Diarrhea
PPPD*	Jaw Click/Pain	Neck Pain	Motion Sensitivity
Sweating	Speech Difficulty	Monthly Cycle	

What time did your symptoms start? ____________

Tinnitus: L R How many noises? ______ Loudness Scale: 1 2 3 4 5

Possible Meniere's Symptom Triggers Today:

Physical: ____________

____

____

____________ Pollen, Mold, Dust, Trees, Grass, Ragweed

Visual: ____________

____

____

Emotional: ____________

____

____

What Helped Me?

Medication/s & Time Taken		Other	
		Prayer	Rest
		Meditation	Friend/s
		Self-care	Family
		Exercise	Pet/s
		Mindfulness	Vestibular Rehab
		Gratitude	Hearing Device

Duration of Vertigo ______ minutes ______ hours ______ days

Severity of Vertigo 1 2 3 4 5 - I HATE you, vertigo!

New Symptoms? ____________

____

What I Accomplished Today – Something to Celebrate! ♡

____

____

____

Three Things I am Thankful for Today:

1.
2.
3.

MONTH: January February March April May June July August September October November December

Day: Monday Tuesday Wednesday Thursday Friday Saturday Sunday

Date: ______ **Season:** Summer Autumn/Fall Winter Spring

Temperature: Low _______ High _______

Barometer: 9am__________ 9pm__________ **Humidity** __________

Sunny	Cloudy	Rain	Showers	Windy
Snow	Storm	Humid	Dry	

Food & Fluid Intake (be mindful of salt):

Breakfast			
Lunch			
Dinner			
Fluid Intake	Water - ______		
Snacks			

Symptoms:

Tinnitus	Vertigo	Drop Attack	Nausea
Anxiety	Brain Fog	Hearing Loss	Hyperacusis
Fatigue	Balance	Co-ordination	Stress
Headache	Migraine	Nystagmus	Disequilibrium
Ear Fullness/ Pressure/Pain	Vision Difficulties	Physical Impairment	Vestibular Migraine
Vomiting	Depression	BPPV*	Diarrhea
PPPD*	Jaw Click/Pain	Neck Pain	Motion Sensitivity
Sweating	Speech Difficulty	Monthly Cycle	

What time did your symptoms start? ____________________

Tinnitus: L R How many noises? ________ Loudness Scale: 1 2 3 4 5

Possible Meniere's Symptom Triggers Today:

Physical: ____________________

____

____

____________________ Pollen, Mold, Dust, Trees, Grass, Ragweed

Visual: ____________________

____

____

Emotional: ____________________

____

____

What Helped Me?

Medication/s & Time Taken		Other	
		Prayer	Rest
		Meditation	Friend/s
		Self-care	Family
		Exercise	Pet/s
		Mindfulness	Vestibular Rehab
		Gratitude	Hearing Device

Duration of Vertigo ________ minutes ________ hours ________ days

Severity of Vertigo 1 2 3 4 5 - I HATE you, vertigo!

New Symptoms? ____________________

____

What I Accomplished Today – Something to Celebrate! ♡

____

____

____

Three Things I am Thankful for Today:

1.
2.
3.

MONTH: January February March April May June July August September October November December

Day: Monday Tuesday Wednesday Thursday Friday Saturday Sunday

Date: ______ **Season:** Summer Autumn/Fall Winter Spring

Temperature: Low ________ High ________

Barometer: 9am__________ 9pm__________ **Humidity** ____________

Sunny	Cloudy	Rain	Showers	Windy
Snow	Storm	Humid	Dry	

Food & Fluid Intake (be mindful of salt):

Breakfast			
Lunch			
Dinner			
Fluid Intake	Water - ______		
Snacks			

Symptoms:

Tinnitus	Vertigo	Drop Attack	Nausea
Anxiety	Brain Fog	Hearing Loss	Hyperacusis
Fatigue	Balance	Co-ordination	Stress
Headache	Migraine	Nystagmus	Disequilibrium
Ear Fullness/ Pressure/Pain	Vision Difficulties	Physical Impairment	Vestibular Migraine
Vomiting	Depression	BPPV*	Diarrhea
PPPD*	Jaw Click/Pain	Neck Pain	Motion Sensitivity
Sweating	Speech Difficulty	Monthly Cycle	

What time did your symptoms start? ____________________

Tinnitus: L R How many noises? ______ Loudness Scale: 1 2 3 4 5

Possible Meniere's Symptom Triggers Today:

Physical: ____________________

____

____

____________________ Pollen, Mold, Dust, Trees, Grass, Ragweed

Visual: ____________________

____

Emotional: ____________________

____

What Helped Me?

Medication/s & Time Taken		Other	
		Prayer	Rest
		Meditation	Friend/s
		Self-care	Family
		Exercise	Pet/s
		Mindfulness	Vestibular Rehab
		Gratitude	Hearing Device

Duration of Vertigo ______ minutes ______ hours ______ days

Severity of Vertigo 1 2 3 4 5 - I HATE you, vertigo!

New Symptoms? ____________________

What I Accomplished Today - Something to Celebrate! ♡

____

____

____

Three Things I am Thankful for Today:

1.
2.
3.

MONTH: January February March April May June July August September October November December

Day: Monday Tuesday Wednesday Thursday Friday Saturday Sunday
Date: ______ **Season:** Summer Autumn/Fall Winter Spring
Temperature: Low _______ High _______
Barometer: 9am__________ 9pm________ **Humidity** ___________

Sunny	Cloudy	Rain	Showers	Windy
Snow	Storm	Humid	Dry	

Food & Fluid Intake (be mindful of salt):

Breakfast			
Lunch			
Dinner			
Fluid Intake	Water - ______		
Snacks			

Symptoms:

Tinnitus	Vertigo	Drop Attack	Nausea
Anxiety	Brain Fog	Hearing Loss	Hyperacusis
Fatigue	Balance	Co-ordination	Stress
Headache	Migraine	Nystagmus	Disequilibrium
Ear Fullness/ Pressure/Pain	Vision Difficulties	Physical Impairment	Vestibular Migraine
Vomiting	Depression	BPPV*	Diarrhea
PPPD*	Jaw Click/Pain	Neck Pain	Motion Sensitivity
Sweating	Speech Difficulty	Monthly Cycle	

What time did your symptoms start? ____________________

Tinnitus: L R How many noises? ______ Loudness Scale: 1 2 3 4 5

Possible Meniere's Symptom Triggers Today:

Physical: ____________________

____

____

____________________ Pollen, Mold, Dust, Trees, Grass, Ragweed

Visual: ____________________

____

____

Emotional: ____________________

____

____

What Helped Me?

Medication/s & Time Taken		Other	
		Prayer	Rest
		Meditation	Friend/s
		Self-care	Family
		Exercise	Pet/s
		Mindfulness	Vestibular Rehab
		Gratitude	Hearing Device

Duration of Vertigo ______ minutes ______ hours______ days

Severity of Vertigo 1 2 3 4 5 - I HATE you, vertigo!

New Symptoms? ____________________

____

What I Accomplished Today - Something to Celebrate! ♡

____

____

____

Three Things I am Thankful for Today:

1.
2.
3.

Vertigo. STOP! There will be a cure! Meniere's disease does not define us. Meniere's, I hate you! Tinnitus. MENIERE'S WARRIOR! Hope – there is always hope! Hearing loss. A cure will be found! Imbalance. Take each day one at a time. BREATHE. Create moments. Find things to be thankful for. Ear pain. You will overcome. Good things are coming. Research. Meniere's, your time is UP! Vertigo. There will be a cure! Meniere's disease does not define us. Meniere's, I hate you! Tinnitus. MENIERE'S WARRIOR! Hope – there is always hope! Hearing loss. A cure will be found! Imbalance. Take each day one at a time. BREATHE. Create moments. Find things to be thankful for. Ear pain. You will overcome. Good things are coming. Research. Meniere's, your time is UP! Vertigo. There will be a cure! Meniere's disease does not define us. Meniere's, I hate you! Tinnitus. MENIERE'S WARRIOR! Hope – there is always hope! Hearing loss. A cure will be found! Imbalance. Take each day one at a time. BREATHE. Create moments. Find things to be thankful for. Ear pain. You will overcome. Good things are coming. Research. Meniere's, your time is UP! Vertigo. There will be a cure! Meniere's disease does not define us. Meniere's, I hate you! Tinnitus. MENIERE'S WARRIOR! Hope, there is always hope! We will be cured! BREATHE...vertigo. STOP! There will be a cure! Meniere's disease does not define us. Meniere's, I hate you! Tinnitus. MENIERE'S WARRIOR! Hope – there is always hope! Hearing loss. A cure will be found! Imbalance. Take each day one at a time. BREATHE. Create moments. Find things to be thankful for. Ear pain. You will overcome. Good things are coming. Research. Meniere's, your time is UP! Vertigo. There will be a cure! Meniere's disease does not define us. Meniere's, I hate you! Tinnitus. MENIERE'S WARRIOR! Hope – there is always hope! Hearing loss. A cure will be found! Imbalance. Take each day one at a time. BREATHE. Create moments. Find things to be thankful for. Ear pain. You will overcome. Good things are coming. Research. Meniere's, your time is UP! Vertigo. There will be a cure! Meniere's disease does not define us. Meniere's, I hate you! Tinnitus. MENIERE'S WARRIOR! Hope – there is always hope! Hearing loss. A cure will be found! Imbalance. Take each day one at a time. BREATHE. Create moments. Find things to be thankful for. Ear pain. You will overcome. Good things are coming. Research. Meniere's, your time is UP! Vertigo. There will be a cure! Meniere's disease does not define us. Meniere's, I hate you! Tinnitus. MENIERE'S WARRIOR! Hope, there is always hope! We will be cured! BREATHE...vertigo. STOP! There will be a cure! Meniere's disease does not define us. Meniere's, I hate you! Tinnitus. MENIERE'S WARRIOR! Hope – there is always hope! Hearing loss. A cure will be found! Imbalance. Take each day one at a time. BREATHE. Create moments. Find things to be thankful for. Ear pain. You will overcome. Good things are coming. Research. Meniere's, your time is UP! Vertigo. **There will be a cure!**

Vertigo. STOP! There will be a cure! Meniere's disease does not define us. Meniere's, I hate you! Tinnitus. MENIERE'S WARRIOR! Hope – there is always hope! Hearing loss. A cure will be found! Imbalance. Take each day one at a time. BREATHE. Create moments. Find things to be thankful for. Ear pain. You will overcome. Good things are coming. Research. Meniere's, your time is UP! Vertigo. There will be a cure! Meniere's disease does not define us. Meniere's, I hate you! Tinnitus. MENIERE'S WARRIOR! Hope – there is always hope! Hearing loss. A cure will be found! Imbalance. Take each day one at a time. BREATHE. Create moments. Find things to be thankful for. Ear pain. You will overcome. Good things are coming. Research. Meniere's, your time is UP! Vertigo. There will be a cure! Meniere's disease does not define us. Meniere's, I hate you! Tinnitus. MENIERE'S WARRIOR! Hope – there is always hope! Hearing loss. A cure will be found! Imbalance. Take each day one at a time. BREATHE. Create moments. Find things to be thankful for. Ear pain. You will overcome. Good things are coming. Research. Meniere's, your time is UP! Vertigo. There will be a cure! Meniere's disease does not define us. Meniere's, I hate you! Tinnitus. MENIERE'S WARRIOR! Hope, there is always hope! We will be cured! BREATHE...vertigo. STOP! There will be a cure! Meniere's disease does not define us. Meniere's, I hate you! Tinnitus. MENIERE'S WARRIOR! Hope – there is always hope! Hearing loss. A cure will be found! Imbalance. Take each day one at a time. BREATHE. Create moments. Find things to be thankful for. Ear pain. You will overcome. Good things are coming. Research. Meniere's, your time is UP! Vertigo. There will be a cure! Meniere's disease does not define us. Meniere's, I hate you! Tinnitus. MENIERE'S WARRIOR! Hope – there is always hope! Hearing loss. A cure will be found! Imbalance. Take each day one at a time. BREATHE. Create moments. Find things to be thankful for. Ear pain. You will overcome. Good things are coming. Research. Meniere's, your time is UP! Vertigo. There will be a cure! Meniere's disease does not define us. Meniere's, I hate you! Tinnitus. MENIERE'S WARRIOR! Hope – there is always hope! Hearing loss. A cure will be found! Imbalance. Take each day one at a time. BREATHE. Create moments. Find things to be thankful for. Ear pain. You will overcome. Good things are coming. Research. Meniere's, your time is UP! Vertigo. There will be a cure! Meniere's disease does not define us. Meniere's, I hate you! Tinnitus. MENIERE'S WARRIOR! Hope, there is always hope! We will be cured! BREATHE...vertigo. STOP! There will be a cure! Meniere's disease does not define us. Meniere's, I hate you! Tinnitus. MENIERE'S WARRIOR! Hope – there is always hope! Hearing loss. A cure will be found! Imbalance. Take each day one at a time. BREATHE. Create moments. Find things to be thankful for. Ear pain. You will overcome. Good things are coming. Research. Meniere's, your time is UP! Vertigo. **There will be a cure!**

MONTH: January February March April May June July August September October November December

Day: Monday Tuesday Wednesday Thursday Friday Saturday Sunday
Date: ______ **Season:** Summer Autumn/Fall Winter Spring
Temperature: Low ______ High ______
Barometer: 9am________ 9pm________ **Humidity** ________

Sunny	Cloudy	Rain	Showers	Windy
Snow	Storm	Humid	Dry	

Food & Fluid Intake (be mindful of salt):

Breakfast			
Lunch			
Dinner			
Fluid Intake	Water - ______		
Snacks			

Symptoms:

Tinnitus	Vertigo	Drop Attack	Nausea
Anxiety	Brain Fog	Hearing Loss	Hyperacusis
Fatigue	Balance	Co-ordination	Stress
Headache	Migraine	Nystagmus	Disequilibrium
Ear Fullness/ Pressure/Pain	Vision Difficulties	Physical Impairment	Vestibular Migraine
Vomiting	Depression	BPPV*	Diarrhea
PPPD*	Jaw Click/Pain	Neck Pain	Motion Sensitivity
Sweating	Speech Difficulty	Monthly Cycle	

What time did your symptoms start? ____________________

Tinnitus: L R How many noises? ______ Loudness Scale: 1 2 3 4 5

Possible Meniere's Symptom Triggers Today:

Physical: ____________________

____

____

____________________ Pollen, Mold, Dust, Trees, Grass, Ragweed

Visual: ____________________

____

Emotional: ____________________

____

____

What Helped Me?

Medication/s & Time Taken		Other	
		Prayer	Rest
		Meditation	Friend/s
		Self-care	Family
		Exercise	Pet/s
		Mindfulness	Vestibular Rehab
		Gratitude	Hearing Device

Duration of Vertigo ______ minutes ______ hours______ days

Severity of Vertigo 1 2 3 4 5 - I HATE you, vertigo!

New Symptoms? ____________________

____

What I Accomplished Today - Something to Celebrate! ♡

____

____

____

Three Things I am Thankful for Today:

1.
2.
3.

MONTH: January February March April May June July August September October November December

Day: Monday Tuesday Wednesday Thursday Friday Saturday Sunday
Date: ______ **Season:** Summer Autumn/Fall Winter Spring
Temperature: Low ______ High ______
Barometer: 9am______ 9pm______ **Humidity** ______

Sunny	Cloudy	Rain	Showers	Windy
Snow	Storm	Humid	Dry	

Food & Fluid Intake (be mindful of salt):

Breakfast			
Lunch			
Dinner			
Fluid Intake	Water - ______		
Snacks			

Symptoms:

Tinnitus	Vertigo	Drop Attack	Nausea
Anxiety	Brain Fog	Hearing Loss	Hyperacusis
Fatigue	Balance	Co-ordination	Stress
Headache	Migraine	Nystagmus	Disequilibrium
Ear Fullness/ Pressure/Pain	Vision Difficulties	Physical Impairment	Vestibular Migraine
Vomiting	Depression	BPPV*	Diarrhea
PPPD*	Jaw Click/Pain	Neck Pain	Motion Sensitivity
Sweating	Speech Difficulty	Monthly Cycle	

What time did your symptoms start? ____________

Tinnitus: L R How many noises? ______ Loudness Scale: 1 2 3 4 5

Possible Meniere's Symptom Triggers Today:

Physical: ____________

____

____

____________ Pollen, Mold, Dust, Trees, Grass, Ragweed

Visual: ____________

____

____

Emotional: ____________

____

____

What Helped Me?

Medication/s & Time Taken		Other	
		Prayer	Rest
		Meditation	Friend/s
		Self-care	Family
		Exercise	Pet/s
		Mindfulness	Vestibular Rehab
		Gratitude	Hearing Device

Duration of Vertigo ______ minutes ______ hours ______ days

Severity of Vertigo 1 2 3 4 5 - I HATE you, vertigo!

New Symptoms? ____________

____

What I Accomplished Today - Something to Celebrate! ♡

____

____

____

Three Things I am Thankful for Today:

1.
2.
3.

MONTH: January February March April May June July August September October November December

Day: Monday Tuesday Wednesday Thursday Friday Saturday Sunday
Date: ______ **Season:** Summer Autumn/Fall Winter Spring
Temperature: Low _______ High _______
Barometer: 9am__________ 9pm__________ **Humidity** ___________

Sunny	Cloudy	Rain	Showers	Windy
Snow	Storm	Humid	Dry	

Food & Fluid Intake (be mindful of salt):

Breakfast			
Lunch			
Dinner			
Fluid Intake	Water - ______		
Snacks			

Symptoms:

Tinnitus	Vertigo	Drop Attack	Nausea
Anxiety	Brain Fog	Hearing Loss	Hyperacusis
Fatigue	Balance	Co-ordination	Stress
Headache	Migraine	Nystagmus	Disequilibrium
Ear Fullness/ Pressure/Pain	Vision Difficulties	Physical Impairment	Vestibular Migraine
Vomiting	Depression	BPPV*	Diarrhea
PPPD*	Jaw Click/Pain	Neck Pain	Motion Sensitivity
Sweating	Speech Difficulty	Monthly Cycle	

What time did your symptoms start? ____________

Tinnitus: L R How many noises? ________ Loudness Scale: 1 2 3 4 5

Possible Meniere's Symptom Triggers Today:

Physical: ____________

____

____

____________ Pollen, Mold, Dust, Trees, Grass, Ragweed

Visual: ____________

____

____

Emotional: ____________

____

____

What Helped Me?

Medication/s & Time Taken		Other	
		Prayer	Rest
		Meditation	Friend/s
		Self-care	Family
		Exercise	Pet/s
		Mindfulness	Vestibular Rehab
		Gratitude	Hearing Device

Duration of Vertigo ______ minutes ______ hours ______ days

Severity of Vertigo 1 2 3 4 5 - I HATE you, vertigo!

New Symptoms? ____________

____

What I Accomplished Today - Something to Celebrate! ♡

____

____

____

Three Things I am Thankful for Today:

1.
2.
3.

MONTH: January February March April May June July August September October November December

Day: Monday Tuesday Wednesday Thursday Friday Saturday Sunday
Date: ______ **Season:** Summer Autumn/Fall Winter Spring
Temperature: Low ______ High ______
Barometer: 9am________ 9pm________ **Humidity** __________

Sunny	Cloudy	Rain	Showers	Windy
Snow	Storm	Humid	Dry	

Food & Fluid Intake (be mindful of salt):

Breakfast			
Lunch			
Dinner			
Fluid Intake	Water - ______		
Snacks			

Symptoms:

Tinnitus	Vertigo	Drop Attack	Nausea
Anxiety	Brain Fog	Hearing Loss	Hyperacusis
Fatigue	Balance	Co-ordination	Stress
Headache	Migraine	Nystagmus	Disequilibrium
Ear Fullness/ Pressure/Pain	Vision Difficulties	Physical Impairment	Vestibular Migraine
Vomiting	Depression	BPPV*	Diarrhea
PPPD*	Jaw Click/Pain	Neck Pain	Motion Sensitivity
Sweating	Speech Difficulty	Monthly Cycle	

What time did your symptoms start? ____________________

Tinnitus: L R How many noises? ______ Loudness Scale: 1 2 3 4 5

Possible Meniere's Symptom Triggers Today:

Physical: ____________________

____

____

____________________ Pollen, Mold, Dust, Trees, Grass, Ragweed

Visual: ____________________

____

____

Emotional: ____________________

____

____

What Helped Me?

Medication/s & Time Taken		Other	
		Prayer	Rest
		Meditation	Friend/s
		Self-care	Family
		Exercise	Pet/s
		Mindfulness	Vestibular Rehab
		Gratitude	Hearing Device

Duration of Vertigo ______ minutes ______ hours ______ days

Severity of Vertigo 1 2 3 4 5 - I HATE you, vertigo!

New Symptoms? ____________________

____

What I Accomplished Today - Something to Celebrate! ♡

____

____

____

Three Things I am Thankful for Today:

1.
2.
3.

MONTH: January February March April May June July August September October November December

Day: Monday Tuesday Wednesday Thursday Friday Saturday Sunday
Date: ______ **Season:** Summer Autumn/Fall Winter Spring
Temperature: Low ______ High ______
Barometer: 9am________ 9pm________ **Humidity** __________

Sunny	Cloudy	Rain	Showers	Windy
Snow	Storm	Humid	Dry	

Food & Fluid Intake (be mindful of salt):

Breakfast			
Lunch			
Dinner			
Fluid Intake	Water - ______		
Snacks			

Symptoms:

Tinnitus	Vertigo	Drop Attack	Nausea
Anxiety	Brain Fog	Hearing Loss	Hyperacusis
Fatigue	Balance	Co-ordination	Stress
Headache	Migraine	Nystagmus	Disequilibrium
Ear Fullness/ Pressure/Pain	Vision Difficulties	Physical Impairment	Vestibular Migraine
Vomiting	Depression	BPPV*	Diarrhea
PPPD*	Jaw Click/Pain	Neck Pain	Motion Sensitivity
Sweating	Speech Difficulty	Monthly Cycle	

What time did your symptoms start? ____________________

Tinnitus: L R How many noises? ______ Loudness Scale: 1 2 3 4 5

Possible Meniere's Symptom Triggers Today:

Physical: ____________________

____

____

____________________ Pollen, Mold, Dust, Trees, Grass, Ragweed

Visual: ____________________

____

____

Emotional: ____________________

____

____

What Helped Me?

Medication/s & Time Taken		Other	
		Prayer	Rest
		Meditation	Friend/s
		Self-care	Family
		Exercise	Pet/s
		Mindfulness	Vestibular Rehab
		Gratitude	Hearing Device

Duration of Vertigo ______ minutes ______ hours ______ days

Severity of Vertigo 1 2 3 4 5 - I HATE you, vertigo!

New Symptoms? ____________________

____

What I Accomplished Today – Something to Celebrate! ♡

____

____

____

Three Things I am Thankful for Today:

1.
2.
3.

MONTH: January February March April May June July August September October November December

Day: Monday Tuesday Wednesday Thursday Friday Saturday Sunday
Date: ______ **Season:** Summer Autumn/Fall Winter Spring
Temperature: Low _______ High _______
Barometer: 9am__________ 9pm__________ **Humidity** ____________

Sunny	Cloudy	Rain	Showers	Windy
Snow	Storm	Humid	Dry	

Food & Fluid Intake (be mindful of salt):

Breakfast			
Lunch			
Dinner			
Fluid Intake	Water - ______		
Snacks			

Symptoms:

Tinnitus	Vertigo	Drop Attack	Nausea
Anxiety	Brain Fog	Hearing Loss	Hyperacusis
Fatigue	Balance	Co-ordination	Stress
Headache	Migraine	Nystagmus	Disequilibrium
Ear Fullness/ Pressure/Pain	Vision Difficulties	Physical Impairment	Vestibular Migraine
Vomiting	Depression	BPPV*	Diarrhea
PPPD*	Jaw Click/Pain	Neck Pain	Motion Sensitivity
Sweating	Speech Difficulty	Monthly Cycle	

What time did your symptoms start? ____________________

Tinnitus: L R How many noises? ________ Loudness Scale: 1 2 3 4 5

Possible Meniere's Symptom Triggers Today:

Physical: ____________________

____

____

____________________ Pollen, Mold, Dust, Trees, Grass, Ragweed

Visual: ____________________

____

____

Emotional: ____________________

____

____

What Helped Me?

Medication/s & Time Taken		Other	
		Prayer	Rest
		Meditation	Friend/s
		Self-care	Family
		Exercise	Pet/s
		Mindfulness	Vestibular Rehab
		Gratitude	Hearing Device

Duration of Vertigo ______ minutes _______ hours______ days

Severity of Vertigo 1 2 3 4 5 - I HATE you, vertigo!

New Symptoms? ____________________

____

What I Accomplished Today – Something to Celebrate! ♡

____

____

____

Three Things I am Thankful for Today:

1.
2.
3.

MONTH: January February March April May June July August September October November December

Day: Monday Tuesday Wednesday Thursday Friday Saturday Sunday
Date: ______ **Season:** Summer Autumn/Fall Winter Spring
Temperature: Low _______ High _______
Barometer: 9am_________ 9pm_________ **Humidity** ___________

Sunny	Cloudy	Rain	Showers	Windy
Snow	Storm	Humid	Dry	

Food & Fluid Intake (be mindful of salt):

Breakfast			
Lunch			
Dinner			
Fluid Intake	Water - ______		
Snacks			

Symptoms:

Tinnitus	Vertigo	Drop Attack	Nausea
Anxiety	Brain Fog	Hearing Loss	Hyperacusis
Fatigue	Balance	Co-ordination	Stress
Headache	Migraine	Nystagmus	Disequilibrium
Ear Fullness/ Pressure/Pain	Vision Difficulties	Physical Impairment	Vestibular Migraine
Vomiting	Depression	BPPV*	Diarrhea
PPPD*	Jaw Click/Pain	Neck Pain	Motion Sensitivity
Sweating	Speech Difficulty	Monthly Cycle	

What time did your symptoms start? ______________________

Tinnitus: L R How many noises? ______ Loudness Scale: 1 2 3 4 5

Possible Meniere's Symptom Triggers Today:

Physical: ____

____

____

______________________ Pollen, Mold, Dust, Trees, Grass, Ragweed

Visual: ____

____

____

Emotional: ____

____

____

What Helped Me?

Medication/s & Time Taken		Other	
		Prayer	Rest
		Meditation	Friend/s
		Self-care	Family
		Exercise	Pet/s
		Mindfulness	Vestibular Rehab
		Gratitude	Hearing Device

Duration of Vertigo ______ minutes ______ hours ______ days

Severity of Vertigo 1 2 3 4 5 - I HATE you, vertigo!

New Symptoms? ______________________________________

____

What I Accomplished Today – Something to Celebrate! ♡

____

____

____

Three Things I am Thankful for Today:

1.
2.
3.

MONTH: January February March April May June July August September October November December

Day: Monday Tuesday Wednesday Thursday Friday Saturday Sunday

Date: ______ **Season:** Summer Autumn/Fall Winter Spring

Temperature: Low _______ High _______

Barometer: 9am________ 9pm________ **Humidity** ____________

Sunny	Cloudy	Rain	Showers	Windy
Snow	Storm	Humid	Dry	

Food & Fluid Intake (be mindful of salt):

Breakfast			
Lunch			
Dinner			
Fluid Intake	Water - ______		
Snacks			

Symptoms:

Tinnitus	Vertigo	Drop Attack	Nausea
Anxiety	Brain Fog	Hearing Loss	Hyperacusis
Fatigue	Balance	Co-ordination	Stress
Headache	Migraine	Nystagmus	Disequilibrium
Ear Fullness/ Pressure/Pain	Vision Difficulties	Physical Impairment	Vestibular Migraine
Vomiting	Depression	BPPV*	Diarrhea
PPPD*	Jaw Click/Pain	Neck Pain	Motion Sensitivity
Sweating	Speech Difficulty	Monthly Cycle	

What time did your symptoms start? ______________________

Tinnitus: L R How many noises? ______ Loudness Scale: 1 2 3 4 5

Possible Meniere's Symptom Triggers Today:

Physical: ____

____

____

______________________ Pollen, Mold, Dust, Trees, Grass, Ragweed

Visual: ____

____

____

Emotional: ____

____

____

What Helped Me?

Medication/s & Time Taken		Other	
		Prayer	Rest
		Meditation	Friend/s
		Self-care	Family
		Exercise	Pet/s
		Mindfulness	Vestibular Rehab
		Gratitude	Hearing Device

Duration of Vertigo ______ minutes ______ hours______ days

Severity of Vertigo 1 2 3 4 5 - I HATE you, vertigo!

New Symptoms? ____

____

What I Accomplished Today - Something to Celebrate! ♡

____

____

____

Three Things I am Thankful for Today:

1.
2.
3.

MONTH: January February March April May June July August September October November December

Day: Monday Tuesday Wednesday Thursday Friday Saturday Sunday
Date: ______ **Season:** Summer Autumn/Fall Winter Spring
Temperature: Low _______ High _______
Barometer: 9am_______ 9pm_______ **Humidity** ___________

Sunny	Cloudy	Rain	Showers	Windy
Snow	Storm	Humid	Dry	

Food & Fluid Intake (be mindful of salt):

Breakfast			
Lunch			
Dinner			
Fluid Intake	Water - _____		
Snacks			

Symptoms:

Tinnitus	Vertigo	Drop Attack	Nausea
Anxiety	Brain Fog	Hearing Loss	Hyperacusis
Fatigue	Balance	Co-ordination	Stress
Headache	Migraine	Nystagmus	Disequilibrium
Ear Fullness/ Pressure/Pain	Vision Difficulties	Physical Impairment	Vestibular Migraine
Vomiting	Depression	BPPV*	Diarrhea
PPPD*	Jaw Click/Pain	Neck Pain	Motion Sensitivity
Sweating	Speech Difficulty	Monthly Cycle	

What time did your symptoms start? ________________

Tinnitus: L R How many noises? _______ Loudness Scale: 1 2 3 4 5

Possible Meniere's Symptom Triggers Today:

Physical: ________________

____

____

________________ Pollen, Mold, Dust, Trees, Grass, Ragweed

Visual: ________________

____

____

Emotional: ________________

____

____

What Helped Me?

Medication/s & Time Taken		Other	
		Prayer	Rest
		Meditation	Friend/s
		Self-care	Family
		Exercise	Pet/s
		Mindfulness	Vestibular Rehab
		Gratitude	Hearing Device

Duration of Vertigo ______ minutes ______ hours______ days

Severity of Vertigo 1 2 3 4 5 - I HATE you, vertigo!

New Symptoms? ________________

____

What I Accomplished Today – Something to Celebrate! ♡

____

____

Three Things I am Thankful for Today:

1.
2.
3.

MONTH: January February March April May June July August September October November December

Day: Monday Tuesday Wednesday Thursday Friday Saturday Sunday
Date: ______ **Season:** Summer Autumn/Fall Winter Spring
Temperature: Low _______ High _______
Barometer: 9am_________ 9pm________ **Humidity** ____________

Sunny	Cloudy	Rain	Showers	Windy
Snow	Storm	Humid	Dry	

Food & Fluid Intake (be mindful of salt):

Breakfast			
Lunch			
Dinner			
Fluid Intake	Water - ______		
Snacks			

Symptoms:

Tinnitus	Vertigo	Drop Attack	Nausea
Anxiety	Brain Fog	Hearing Loss	Hyperacusis
Fatigue	Balance	Co-ordination	Stress
Headache	Migraine	Nystagmus	Disequilibrium
Ear Fullness/ Pressure/Pain	Vision Difficulties	Physical Impairment	Vestibular Migraine
Vomiting	Depression	BPPV*	Diarrhea
PPPD*	Jaw Click/Pain	Neck Pain	Motion Sensitivity
Sweating	Speech Difficulty	Monthly Cycle	

What time did your symptoms start? ______________________

Tinnitus: L R How many noises? ______ Loudness Scale: 1 2 3 4 5

Possible Meniere's Symptom Triggers Today:

Physical: ____

____

____

______________________ Pollen, Mold, Dust, Trees, Grass, Ragweed

Visual: ____

____

____

Emotional: ____

____

____

What Helped Me?

Medication/s & Time Taken		Other	
		Prayer	Rest
		Meditation	Friend/s
		Self-care	Family
		Exercise	Pet/s
		Mindfulness	Vestibular Rehab
		Gratitude	Hearing Device

Duration of Vertigo ______ minutes ______ hours ______ days

Severity of Vertigo 1 2 3 4 5 - I HATE you, vertigo!

New Symptoms? ____

____

What I Accomplished Today – Something to Celebrate! ♡

____

____

____

Three Things I am Thankful for Today:

1.
2.
3.

MONTH: January February March April May June July August September October November December

Day: Monday Tuesday Wednesday Thursday Friday Saturday Sunday

Date: ______ Season: Summer Autumn/Fall Winter Spring

Temperature: Low ______ High ______

Barometer: 9am______ 9pm______ **Humidity** ______

Sunny	Cloudy	Rain	Showers	Windy
Snow	Storm	Humid	Dry	

Food & Fluid Intake (be mindful of salt):

Breakfast			
Lunch			
Dinner			
Fluid Intake	Water - ______		
Snacks			

Symptoms:

Tinnitus	Vertigo	Drop Attack	Nausea
Anxiety	Brain Fog	Hearing Loss	Hyperacusis
Fatigue	Balance	Co-ordination	Stress
Headache	Migraine	Nystagmus	Disequilibrium
Ear Fullness/ Pressure/Pain	Vision Difficulties	Physical Impairment	Vestibular Migraine
Vomiting	Depression	BPPV*	Diarrhea
PPPD*	Jaw Click/Pain	Neck Pain	Motion Sensitivity
Sweating	Speech Difficulty	Monthly Cycle	

What time did your symptoms start? ______________________

Tinnitus: L R How many noises? ______ Loudness Scale: 1 2 3 4 5

Possible Meniere's Symptom Triggers Today:

Physical: ______________________

____

____

______________________ Pollen, Mold, Dust, Trees, Grass, Ragweed

Visual: ______________________

____

____

Emotional: ______________________

____

____

What Helped Me?

Medication/s & Time Taken		Other	
		Prayer	Rest
		Meditation	Friend/s
		Self-care	Family
		Exercise	Pet/s
		Mindfulness	Vestibular Rehab
		Gratitude	Hearing Device

Duration of Vertigo ______ minutes ______ hours ______ days

Severity of Vertigo 1 2 3 4 5 - I HATE you, vertigo!

New Symptoms? ______________________

____

What I Accomplished Today – Something to Celebrate! ♡

____

____

____

Three Things I am Thankful for Today:

1.
2.
3.

MONTH: January February March April May June July August September October November December

Day: Monday Tuesday Wednesday Thursday Friday Saturday Sunday
Date: ______ **Season:** Summer Autumn/Fall Winter Spring
Temperature: Low _______ High _______
Barometer: 9am________ 9pm________ **Humidity** ____________

Sunny	Cloudy	Rain	Showers	Windy
Snow	Storm	Humid	Dry	

Food & Fluid Intake (be mindful of salt):

Breakfast			
Lunch			
Dinner			
Fluid Intake	Water - ______		
Snacks			

Symptoms:

Tinnitus	Vertigo	Drop Attack	Nausea
Anxiety	Brain Fog	Hearing Loss	Hyperacusis
Fatigue	Balance	Co-ordination	Stress
Headache	Migraine	Nystagmus	Disequilibrium
Ear Fullness/ Pressure/Pain	Vision Difficulties	Physical Impairment	Vestibular Migraine
Vomiting	Depression	BPPV*	Diarrhea
PPPD*	Jaw Click/Pain	Neck Pain	Motion Sensitivity
Sweating	Speech Difficulty	Monthly Cycle	

What time did your symptoms start? ______________

Tinnitus: L R How many noises? _______ Loudness Scale: 1 2 3 4 5

Possible Meniere's Symptom Triggers Today:

Physical: ______________

____

____

______________ Pollen, Mold, Dust, Trees, Grass, Ragweed

Visual: ______________

____

____

Emotional: ______________

____

____

What Helped Me?

Medication/s & Time Taken		Other	
		Prayer	Rest
		Meditation	Friend/s
		Self-care	Family
		Exercise	Pet/s
		Mindfulness	Vestibular Rehab
		Gratitude	Hearing Device

Duration of Vertigo ______ minutes ______ hours______ days

Severity of Vertigo 1 2 3 4 5 - I HATE you, vertigo!

New Symptoms? ______________

____

What I Accomplished Today – Something to Celebrate! ♡

____

____

____

Three Things I am Thankful for Today:

1.
2.
3.

MONTH: January February March April May June July August September October November December

Day: Monday Tuesday Wednesday Thursday Friday Saturday Sunday
Date: ______ **Season:** Summer Autumn/Fall Winter Spring
Temperature: Low _______ High _______
Barometer: 9am__________ 9pm_________ **Humidity** ____________

Sunny	Cloudy	Rain	Showers	Windy
Snow	Storm	Humid	Dry	

Food & Fluid Intake (be mindful of salt):

Breakfast			
Lunch			
Dinner			
Fluid Intake	Water - ______		
Snacks			

Symptoms:

Tinnitus	Vertigo	Drop Attack	Nausea
Anxiety	Brain Fog	Hearing Loss	Hyperacusis
Fatigue	Balance	Co-ordination	Stress
Headache	Migraine	Nystagmus	Disequilibrium
Ear Fullness/ Pressure/Pain	Vision Difficulties	Physical Impairment	Vestibular Migraine
Vomiting	Depression	BPPV*	Diarrhea
PPPD*	Jaw Click/Pain	Neck Pain	Motion Sensitivity
Sweating	Speech Difficulty	Monthly Cycle	

What time did your symptoms start? ____________________

Tinnitus: L R How many noises? ______ Loudness Scale: 1 2 3 4 5

Possible Meniere's Symptom Triggers Today:

Physical: ____________________

____

____

____________________ Pollen, Mold, Dust, Trees, Grass, Ragweed

Visual: ____________________

____

____

Emotional: ____________________

____

____

What Helped Me?

Medication/s & Time Taken		Other	
		Prayer	Rest
		Meditation	Friend/s
		Self-care	Family
		Exercise	Pet/s
		Mindfulness	Vestibular Rehab
		Gratitude	Hearing Device

Duration of Vertigo ______ minutes ______ hours ______ days

Severity of Vertigo 1 2 3 4 5 - I HATE you, vertigo!

New Symptoms? ____________________

____

What I Accomplished Today - Something to Celebrate! ♡

____

____

____

Three Things I am Thankful for Today:

1.
2.
3.

MONTH: January February March April May June July August September October November December

Day: Monday Tuesday Wednesday Thursday Friday Saturday Sunday

Date: ______ **Season:** Summer Autumn/Fall Winter Spring

Temperature: Low _______ High _______

Barometer: 9am__________ 9pm_______ **Humidity** __________

Sunny	Cloudy	Rain	Showers	Windy
Snow	Storm	Humid	Dry	

Food & Fluid Intake (be mindful of salt):

Breakfast			
Lunch			
Dinner			
Fluid Intake	Water - ______		
Snacks			

Symptoms:

Tinnitus	Vertigo	Drop Attack	Nausea
Anxiety	Brain Fog	Hearing Loss	Hyperacusis
Fatigue	Balance	Co-ordination	Stress
Headache	Migraine	Nystagmus	Disequilibrium
Ear Fullness/ Pressure/Pain	Vision Difficulties	Physical Impairment	Vestibular Migraine
Vomiting	Depression	BPPV*	Diarrhea
PPPD*	Jaw Click/Pain	Neck Pain	Motion Sensitivity
Sweating	Speech Difficulty	Monthly Cycle	

What time did your symptoms start? ______________________

Tinnitus: L R How many noises? ______ Loudness Scale: 1 2 3 4 5

Possible Meniere's Symptom Triggers Today:

Physical: ______________________

____

____

______________________ Pollen, Mold, Dust, Trees, Grass, Ragweed

Visual: ______________________

____

____

Emotional: ______________________

____

____

What Helped Me?

Medication/s & Time Taken		Other	
		Prayer	Rest
		Meditation	Friend/s
		Self-care	Family
		Exercise	Pet/s
		Mindfulness	Vestibular Rehab
		Gratitude	Hearing Device

Duration of Vertigo ______ minutes ______ hours______ days

Severity of Vertigo 1 2 3 4 5 - I HATE you, vertigo!

New Symptoms? ______________________

____

What I Accomplished Today - Something to Celebrate! ♡

____

____

____

Three Things I am Thankful for Today:

1.
2.
3.

MONTH: January February March April May June July August September October November December

Day: Monday Tuesday Wednesday Thursday Friday Saturday Sunday
Date: ______ **Season:** Summer Autumn/Fall Winter Spring
Temperature: Low ______ High ______
Barometer: 9am______ 9pm______ **Humidity** ________

Sunny	Cloudy	Rain	Showers	Windy
Snow	Storm	Humid	Dry	

Food & Fluid Intake (be mindful of salt):

Breakfast			
Lunch			
Dinner			
Fluid Intake	Water - ______		
Snacks			

Symptoms:

Tinnitus	Vertigo	Drop Attack	Nausea
Anxiety	Brain Fog	Hearing Loss	Hyperacusis
Fatigue	Balance	Co-ordination	Stress
Headache	Migraine	Nystagmus	Disequilibrium
Ear Fullness/ Pressure/Pain	Vision Difficulties	Physical Impairment	Vestibular Migraine
Vomiting	Depression	BPPV*	Diarrhea
PPPD*	Jaw Click/Pain	Neck Pain	Motion Sensitivity
Sweating	Speech Difficulty	Monthly Cycle	

What time did your symptoms start? ____________

Tinnitus: L R How many noises? ______ Loudness Scale: 1 2 3 4 5

Possible Meniere's Symptom Triggers Today:

Physical: ____________

____

____

____________ Pollen, Mold, Dust, Trees, Grass, Ragweed

Visual: ____________

____

____

Emotional: ____________

____

____

What Helped Me?

Medication/s & Time Taken		Other	
		Prayer	Rest
		Meditation	Friend/s
		Self-care	Family
		Exercise	Pet/s
		Mindfulness	Vestibular Rehab
		Gratitude	Hearing Device

Duration of Vertigo ______ minutes ______ hours ______ days

Severity of Vertigo 1 2 3 4 5 - I HATE you, vertigo!

New Symptoms? ____________

____

What I Accomplished Today - Something to Celebrate! ♡

____

____

____

Three Things I am Thankful for Today:

1.
2.
3.

MONTH: January February March April May June July August September October November December

Day: Monday Tuesday Wednesday Thursday Friday Saturday Sunday
Date: ______ **Season:** Summer Autumn/Fall Winter Spring
Temperature: Low _______ High _______
Barometer: 9am_________ 9pm________ **Humidity** ____________

Sunny	Cloudy	Rain	Showers	Windy
Snow	Storm	Humid	Dry	

Food & Fluid Intake (be mindful of salt):

Breakfast			
Lunch			
Dinner			
Fluid Intake	Water - ______		
Snacks			

Symptoms:

Tinnitus	Vertigo	Drop Attack	Nausea
Anxiety	Brain Fog	Hearing Loss	Hyperacusis
Fatigue	Balance	Co-ordination	Stress
Headache	Migraine	Nystagmus	Disequilibrium
Ear Fullness/ Pressure/Pain	Vision Difficulties	Physical Impairment	Vestibular Migraine
Vomiting	Depression	BPPV*	Diarrhea
PPPD*	Jaw Click/Pain	Neck Pain	Motion Sensitivity
Sweating	Speech Difficulty	Monthly Cycle	

What time did your symptoms start? ______________

Tinnitus: L R How many noises? ______ Loudness Scale: 1 2 3 4 5

Possible Meniere's Symptom Triggers Today:

Physical: ____

____

____

______________________ Pollen, Mold, Dust, Trees, Grass, Ragweed

Visual: ____

____

Emotional: ____

____

____

What Helped Me?

Medication/s & Time Taken		Other	
		Prayer	Rest
		Meditation	Friend/s
		Self-care	Family
		Exercise	Pet/s
		Mindfulness	Vestibular Rehab
		Gratitude	Hearing Device

Duration of Vertigo ______ minutes ______ hours ______ days

Severity of Vertigo 1 2 3 4 5 - I HATE you, vertigo!

New Symptoms? ____

____

What I Accomplished Today - Something to Celebrate! ♡

____

____

____

Three Things I am Thankful for Today:

1.
2.
3.

MONTH: January February March April May June July August September October November December

Day: Monday Tuesday Wednesday Thursday Friday Saturday Sunday

Date: ______ **Season:** Summer Autumn/Fall Winter Spring

Temperature: Low ______ High ______

Barometer: 9am______ 9pm______ **Humidity** ____________

Sunny	Cloudy	Rain	Showers	Windy
Snow	Storm	Humid	Dry	

Food & Fluid Intake (be mindful of salt):

Breakfast			
Lunch			
Dinner			
Fluid Intake	Water - ______		
Snacks			

Symptoms:

Tinnitus	Vertigo	Drop Attack	Nausea
Anxiety	Brain Fog	Hearing Loss	Hyperacusis
Fatigue	Balance	Co-ordination	Stress
Headache	Migraine	Nystagmus	Disequilibrium
Ear Fullness/ Pressure/Pain	Vision Difficulties	Physical Impairment	Vestibular Migraine
Vomiting	Depression	BPPV*	Diarrhea
PPPD*	Jaw Click/Pain	Neck Pain	Motion Sensitivity
Sweating	Speech Difficulty	Monthly Cycle	

What time did your symptoms start? ____________________

Tinnitus: L R How many noises? ______ Loudness Scale: 1 2 3 4 5

Possible Meniere's Symptom Triggers Today:

Physical:____

____

____

____________________ Pollen, Mold, Dust, Trees, Grass, Ragweed

Visual: ____

____

Emotional: ____

____

____

What Helped Me?

Medication/s & Time Taken		Other	
		Prayer	Rest
		Meditation	Friend/s
		Self-care	Family
		Exercise	Pet/s
		Mindfulness	Vestibular Rehab
		Gratitude	Hearing Device

Duration of Vertigo ______ minutes ______ hours ______ days

Severity of Vertigo 1 2 3 4 5 - I HATE you, vertigo!

New Symptoms? ____

____

What I Accomplished Today – Something to Celebrate! ♡

____

____

____

Three Things I am Thankful for Today:

1.
2.
3.

MONTH: January February March April May June July August September October November December

Day: Monday Tuesday Wednesday Thursday Friday Saturday Sunday
Date: ______ **Season:** Summer Autumn/Fall Winter Spring
Temperature: Low _______ High _______
Barometer: 9am_______ 9pm_______ **Humidity** ___________

Sunny	Cloudy	Rain	Showers	Windy
Snow	Storm	Humid	Dry	

Food & Fluid Intake (be mindful of salt):

Breakfast			
Lunch			
Dinner			
Fluid Intake	Water - ______		
Snacks			

Symptoms:

Tinnitus	Vertigo	Drop Attack	Nausea
Anxiety	Brain Fog	Hearing Loss	Hyperacusis
Fatigue	Balance	Co-ordination	Stress
Headache	Migraine	Nystagmus	Disequilibrium
Ear Fullness/ Pressure/Pain	Vision Difficulties	Physical Impairment	Vestibular Migraine
Vomiting	Depression	BPPV*	Diarrhea
PPPD*	Jaw Click/Pain	Neck Pain	Motion Sensitivity
Sweating	Speech Difficulty	Monthly Cycle	

What time did your symptoms start? ______________________

Tinnitus: L R How many noises? ________ Loudness Scale: 1 2 3 4 5

Possible Meniere's Symptom Triggers Today:

Physical: ____

____

____

______________________ Pollen, Mold, Dust, Trees, Grass, Ragweed

Visual: ____

____

____

Emotional: ____

____

____

What Helped Me?

Medication/s & Time Taken		Other	
		Prayer	Rest
		Meditation	Friend/s
		Self-care	Family
		Exercise	Pet/s
		Mindfulness	Vestibular Rehab
		Gratitude	Hearing Device

Duration of Vertigo _______ minutes ________ hours______ days

Severity of Vertigo 1 2 3 4 5 - I HATE you, vertigo!

New Symptoms? ____

____

What I Accomplished Today - Something to Celebrate! ♡

____

____

____

Three Things I am Thankful for Today:

1.
2.
3.

MONTH: January February March April May June July August September October November December

Day: Monday Tuesday Wednesday Thursday Friday Saturday Sunday
Date: ______ **Season:** Summer Autumn/Fall Winter Spring
Temperature: Low ________ High ________
Barometer: 9am__________ 9pm_________ **Humidity** ____________

Sunny	Cloudy	Rain	Showers	Windy
Snow	Storm	Humid	Dry	

Food & Fluid Intake (be mindful of salt):

Breakfast			
Lunch			
Dinner			
Fluid Intake	Water -		
Snacks			

Symptoms:

Tinnitus	Vertigo	Drop Attack	Nausea
Anxiety	Brain Fog	Hearing Loss	Hyperacusis
Fatigue	Balance	Co-ordination	Stress
Headache	Migraine	Nystagmus	Disequilibrium
Ear Fullness/ Pressure/Pain	Vision Difficulties	Physical Impairment	Vestibular Migraine
Vomiting	Depression	BPPV*	Diarrhea
PPPD*	Jaw Click/Pain	Neck Pain	Motion Sensitivity
Sweating	Speech Difficulty	Monthly Cycle	

What time did your symptoms start? ____________

Tinnitus: L R How many noises? ______ Loudness Scale: 1 2 3 4 5

Possible Meniere's Symptom Triggers Today:

Physical: ____________

____

____

____________ Pollen, Mold, Dust, Trees, Grass, Ragweed

Visual: ____________

____

Emotional: ____________

____

____

What Helped Me?

Medication/s & Time Taken		Other	
		Prayer	Rest
		Meditation	Friend/s
		Self-care	Family
		Exercise	Pet/s
		Mindfulness	Vestibular Rehab
		Gratitude	Hearing Device

Duration of Vertigo ______ minutes ______ hours______ days

Severity of Vertigo 1 2 3 4 5 - I HATE you, vertigo!

New Symptoms? ____________

____

What I Accomplished Today – Something to Celebrate! ♡

____

____

____

Three Things I am Thankful for Today:

1.
2.
3.

MONTH: January February March April May June July August September October November December

Day: Monday Tuesday Wednesday Thursday Friday Saturday Sunday
Date: ______ **Season:** Summer Autumn/Fall Winter Spring
Temperature: Low _______ High _______
Barometer: 9am__________ 9pm__________ **Humidity** ___________

Sunny	Cloudy	Rain	Showers	Windy
Snow	Storm	Humid	Dry	

Food & Fluid Intake (be mindful of salt):

Breakfast			
Lunch			
Dinner			
Fluid Intake	Water - ____		
Snacks			

Symptoms:

Tinnitus	Vertigo	Drop Attack	Nausea
Anxiety	Brain Fog	Hearing Loss	Hyperacusis
Fatigue	Balance	Co-ordination	Stress
Headache	Migraine	Nystagmus	Disequilibrium
Ear Fullness/ Pressure/Pain	Vision Difficulties	Physical Impairment	Vestibular Migraine
Vomiting	Depression	BPPV*	Diarrhea
PPPD*	Jaw Click/Pain	Neck Pain	Motion Sensitivity
Sweating	Speech Difficulty	Monthly Cycle	

What time did your symptoms start? ____________________

Tinnitus: L R How many noises? ______ Loudness Scale: 1 2 3 4 5

Possible Meniere's Symptom Triggers Today:

Physical: ____________________

____

____

____________________ Pollen, Mold, Dust, Trees, Grass, Ragweed

Visual: ____________________

____

____

Emotional: ____________________

____

____

What Helped Me?

Medication/s & Time Taken		Other	
		Prayer	Rest
		Meditation	Friend/s
		Self-care	Family
		Exercise	Pet/s
		Mindfulness	Vestibular Rehab
		Gratitude	Hearing Device

Duration of Vertigo ______ minutes ______ hours ______ days

Severity of Vertigo 1 2 3 4 5 - I HATE you, vertigo!

New Symptoms? ____________________

____

What I Accomplished Today – Something to Celebrate! ♡

____

____

____

Three Things I am Thankful for Today:

1.
2.
3.

MONTH: January February March April May June July August September October November December

Day: Monday Tuesday Wednesday Thursday Friday Saturday Sunday

Date: ______ **Season:** Summer Autumn/Fall Winter Spring

Temperature: Low ______ High ______

Barometer: 9am______ 9pm______ **Humidity** __________

Sunny	Cloudy	Rain	Showers	Windy
Snow	Storm	Humid	Dry	

Food & Fluid Intake (be mindful of salt):

Breakfast			
Lunch			
Dinner			
Fluid Intake	Water - ______		
Snacks			

Symptoms:

Tinnitus	Vertigo	Drop Attack	Nausea
Anxiety	Brain Fog	Hearing Loss	Hyperacusis
Fatigue	Balance	Co-ordination	Stress
Headache	Migraine	Nystagmus	Disequilibrium
Ear Fullness/ Pressure/Pain	Vision Difficulties	Physical Impairment	Vestibular Migraine
Vomiting	Depression	BPPV*	Diarrhea
PPPD*	Jaw Click/Pain	Neck Pain	Motion Sensitivity
Sweating	Speech Difficulty	Monthly Cycle	

What time did your symptoms start? ____________

Tinnitus: L R How many noises? ______ Loudness Scale: 1 2 3 4 5

Possible Meniere's Symptom Triggers Today:

Physical: ____________

Pollen, Mold, Dust, Trees, Grass, Ragweed

Visual: ____________

Emotional: ____________

What Helped Me?

Medication/s & Time Taken		Other	
		Prayer	Rest
		Meditation	Friend/s
		Self-care	Family
		Exercise	Pet/s
		Mindfulness	Vestibular Rehab
		Gratitude	Hearing Device

Duration of Vertigo ______ minutes ______ hours ______ days

Severity of Vertigo 1 2 3 4 5 - I HATE you, vertigo!

New Symptoms? ____________

What I Accomplished Today – Something to Celebrate! ♡

Three Things I am Thankful for Today:

1.
2.
3.

MONTH: January February March April May June July August September October November December

Day: Monday Tuesday Wednesday Thursday Friday Saturday Sunday

Date: ______ **Season:** Summer Autumn/Fall Winter Spring

Temperature: Low ________ High ________

Barometer: 9am__________ 9pm__________ **Humidity** ____________

Sunny	Cloudy	Rain	Showers	Windy
Snow	Storm	Humid	Dry	

Food & Fluid Intake (be mindful of salt):

Breakfast			
Lunch			
Dinner			
Fluid Intake	Water - ______		
Snacks			

Symptoms:

Tinnitus	Vertigo	Drop Attack	Nausea
Anxiety	Brain Fog	Hearing Loss	Hyperacusis
Fatigue	Balance	Co-ordination	Stress
Headache	Migraine	Nystagmus	Disequilibrium
Ear Fullness/ Pressure/Pain	Vision Difficulties	Physical Impairment	Vestibular Migraine
Vomiting	Depression	BPPV*	Diarrhea
PPPD*	Jaw Click/Pain	Neck Pain	Motion Sensitivity
Sweating	Speech Difficulty	Monthly Cycle	

What time did your symptoms start? ____________________

Tinnitus: L R How many noises? ______ Loudness Scale: 1 2 3 4 5

Possible Meniere's Symptom Triggers Today:

Physical: ____________________

____

____

____________________ Pollen, Mold, Dust, Trees, Grass, Ragweed

Visual: ____________________

____

Emotional: ____________________

____

____

What Helped Me?

Medication/s & Time Taken		Other	
		Prayer	Rest
		Meditation	Friend/s
		Self-care	Family
		Exercise	Pet/s
		Mindfulness	Vestibular Rehab
		Gratitude	Hearing Device

Duration of Vertigo ______ minutes ______ hours ______ days

Severity of Vertigo 1 2 3 4 5 - I HATE you, vertigo!

New Symptoms? ____________________

____

What I Accomplished Today - Something to Celebrate! ♡

____

____

____

Three Things I am Thankful for Today:

1.
2.
3.

MONTH: January February March April May June July August September October November December

Day: Monday Tuesday Wednesday Thursday Friday Saturday Sunday
Date: ______ **Season:** Summer Autumn/Fall Winter Spring
Temperature: Low ______ High ______
Barometer: 9am ______ 9pm ______ **Humidity** ______

Sunny	Cloudy	Rain	Showers	Windy
Snow	Storm	Humid	Dry	

Food & Fluid Intake (be mindful of salt):

Breakfast			
Lunch			
Dinner			
Fluid Intake	Water - ______		
Snacks			

Symptoms:

Tinnitus	Vertigo	Drop Attack	Nausea
Anxiety	Brain Fog	Hearing Loss	Hyperacusis
Fatigue	Balance	Co-ordination	Stress
Headache	Migraine	Nystagmus	Disequilibrium
Ear Fullness/ Pressure/Pain	Vision Difficulties	Physical Impairment	Vestibular Migraine
Vomiting	Depression	BPPV*	Diarrhea
PPPD*	Jaw Click/Pain	Neck Pain	Motion Sensitivity
Sweating	Speech Difficulty	Monthly Cycle	

What time did your symptoms start? ______________________

Tinnitus: L R How many noises? ________ Loudness Scale: 1 2 3 4 5

Possible Meniere's Symptom Triggers Today:

Physical: ______________________

____

____

______________________ Pollen, Mold, Dust, Trees, Grass, Ragweed

Visual: ______________________

____

Emotional: ______________________

____

____

What Helped Me?

Medication/s & Time Taken		Other	
		Prayer	Rest
		Meditation	Friend/s
		Self-care	Family
		Exercise	Pet/s
		Mindfulness	Vestibular Rehab
		Gratitude	Hearing Device

Duration of Vertigo _______ minutes _______ hours______ days

Severity of Vertigo 1 2 3 4 5 - I HATE you, vertigo!

New Symptoms? ______________________

____

What I Accomplished Today – Something to Celebrate! ♡

____

____

____

Three Things I am Thankful for Today:

1.
2.
3.

MONTH: January February March April May June July August September October November December

Day: Monday Tuesday Wednesday Thursday Friday Saturday Sunday
Date: ______ **Season:** Summer Autumn/Fall Winter Spring
Temperature: Low ______ High ______
Barometer: 9am______ 9pm______ **Humidity** ___________

Sunny	Cloudy	Rain	Showers	Windy
Snow	Storm	Humid	Dry	

Food & Fluid Intake (be mindful of salt):

Breakfast			
Lunch			
Dinner			
Fluid Intake	Water - ______		
Snacks			

Symptoms:

Tinnitus	Vertigo	Drop Attack	Nausea
Anxiety	Brain Fog	Hearing Loss	Hyperacusis
Fatigue	Balance	Co-ordination	Stress
Headache	Migraine	Nystagmus	Disequilibrium
Ear Fullness/ Pressure/Pain	Vision Difficulties	Physical Impairment	Vestibular Migraine
Vomiting	Depression	BPPV*	Diarrhea
PPPD*	Jaw Click/Pain	Neck Pain	Motion Sensitivity
Sweating	Speech Difficulty	Monthly Cycle	

What time did your symptoms start? ____________

Tinnitus: L R How many noises? ______ Loudness Scale: 1 2 3 4 5

Possible Meniere's Symptom Triggers Today:

Physical: ____________

____________ Pollen, Mold, Dust, Trees, Grass, Ragweed

Visual: ____________

Emotional: ____________

What Helped Me?

Medication/s & Time Taken		Other	
		Prayer	Rest
		Meditation	Friend/s
		Self-care	Family
		Exercise	Pet/s
		Mindfulness	Vestibular Rehab
		Gratitude	Hearing Device

Duration of Vertigo ______ minutes ______ hours ______ days

Severity of Vertigo 1 2 3 4 5 - I HATE you, vertigo!

New Symptoms? ____________

What I Accomplished Today – Something to Celebrate! ♡

Three Things I am Thankful for Today:

1.
2.
3.

MONTH: January February March April May June July August September October November December

Day: Monday Tuesday Wednesday Thursday Friday Saturday Sunday
Date: ______ **Season:** Summer Autumn/Fall Winter Spring
Temperature: Low _______ High _______
Barometer: 9am_________ 9pm________ **Humidity** ____________

Sunny	Cloudy	Rain	Showers	Windy
Snow	Storm	Humid	Dry	

Food & Fluid Intake (be mindful of salt):

Breakfast			
Lunch			
Dinner			
Fluid Intake	Water - ____		
Snacks			

Symptoms:

Tinnitus	Vertigo	Drop Attack	Nausea
Anxiety	Brain Fog	Hearing Loss	Hyperacusis
Fatigue	Balance	Co-ordination	Stress
Headache	Migraine	Nystagmus	Disequilibrium
Ear Fullness/ Pressure/Pain	Vision Difficulties	Physical Impairment	Vestibular Migraine
Vomiting	Depression	BPPV*	Diarrhea
PPPD*	Jaw Click/Pain	Neck Pain	Motion Sensitivity
Sweating	Speech Difficulty	Monthly Cycle	

What time did your symptoms start? ____________

Tinnitus: L R How many noises? ______ Loudness Scale: 1 2 3 4 5

Possible Meniere's Symptom Triggers Today:

Physical: ____________

____

____

____________ Pollen, Mold, Dust, Trees, Grass, Ragweed

Visual: ____________

____

____

Emotional: ____________

____

____

What Helped Me?

Medication/s & Time Taken		Other	
		Prayer	Rest
		Meditation	Friend/s
		Self-care	Family
		Exercise	Pet/s
		Mindfulness	Vestibular Rehab
		Gratitude	Hearing Device

Duration of Vertigo ______ minutes ______ hours ______ days

Severity of Vertigo 1 2 3 4 5 - I HATE you, vertigo!

New Symptoms? ____________

____

What I Accomplished Today – Something to Celebrate! ♡

____

____

____

Three Things I am Thankful for Today:

1.
2.
3.

MONTH: January February March April May June July August September October November December

Day: Monday Tuesday Wednesday Thursday Friday Saturday Sunday
Date: ______ **Season:** Summer Autumn/Fall Winter Spring
Temperature: Low ______ High ______
Barometer: 9am________ 9pm________ **Humidity** ________

Sunny	Cloudy	Rain	Showers	Windy
Snow	Storm	Humid	Dry	

Food & Fluid Intake (be mindful of salt):

Breakfast			
Lunch			
Dinner			
Fluid Intake	Water - ______		
Snacks			

Symptoms:

Tinnitus	Vertigo	Drop Attack	Nausea
Anxiety	Brain Fog	Hearing Loss	Hyperacusis
Fatigue	Balance	Co-ordination	Stress
Headache	Migraine	Nystagmus	Disequilibrium
Ear Fullness/ Pressure/Pain	Vision Difficulties	Physical Impairment	Vestibular Migraine
Vomiting	Depression	BPPV*	Diarrhea
PPPD*	Jaw Click/Pain	Neck Pain	Motion Sensitivity
Sweating	Speech Difficulty	Monthly Cycle	

What time did your symptoms start? ____________________

Tinnitus: L R How many noises? _______ Loudness Scale: 1 2 3 4 5

Possible Meniere's Symptom Triggers Today:

Physical: ____

____

____

____________________ Pollen, Mold, Dust, Trees, Grass, Ragweed

Visual: ____

____

____

Emotional: ____

____

____

What Helped Me?

Medication/s & Time Taken		Other	
		Prayer	Rest
		Meditation	Friend/s
		Self-care	Family
		Exercise	Pet/s
		Mindfulness	Vestibular Rehab
		Gratitude	Hearing Device

Duration of Vertigo ______ minutes ______ hours ______ days

Severity of Vertigo 1 2 3 4 5 - I HATE you, vertigo!

New Symptoms? ____

____

What I Accomplished Today - Something to Celebrate! ♡

____

____

____

Three Things I am Thankful for Today:

1.
2.
3.

MONTH: January February March April May June July August September October November December

Day: Monday Tuesday Wednesday Thursday Friday Saturday Sunday

Date: ______ **Season:** Summer Autumn/Fall Winter Spring

Temperature: Low ______ High ______

Barometer: 9am______ 9pm______ **Humidity** ______

Sunny	Cloudy	Rain	Showers	Windy
Snow	Storm	Humid	Dry	

Food & Fluid Intake (be mindful of salt):

Breakfast			
Lunch			
Dinner			
Fluid Intake	Water - ______		
Snacks			

Symptoms:

Tinnitus	Vertigo	Drop Attack	Nausea
Anxiety	Brain Fog	Hearing Loss	Hyperacusis
Fatigue	Balance	Co-ordination	Stress
Headache	Migraine	Nystagmus	Disequilibrium
Ear Fullness/ Pressure/Pain	Vision Difficulties	Physical Impairment	Vestibular Migraine
Vomiting	Depression	BPPV*	Diarrhea
PPPD*	Jaw Click/Pain	Neck Pain	Motion Sensitivity
Sweating	Speech Difficulty	Monthly Cycle	

What time did your symptoms start? ______________

Tinnitus: L R How many noises? ________ Loudness Scale: 1 2 3 4 5

Possible Meniere's Symptom Triggers Today:

Physical: ______________

____

____

______________ Pollen, Mold, Dust, Trees, Grass, Ragweed

Visual: ______________

____

____

Emotional: ______________

____

____

What Helped Me?

Medication/s & Time Taken		Other	
		Prayer	Rest
		Meditation	Friend/s
		Self-care	Family
		Exercise	Pet/s
		Mindfulness	Vestibular Rehab
		Gratitude	Hearing Device

Duration of Vertigo ______ minutes ______ hours______ days

Severity of Vertigo 1 2 3 4 5 - I HATE you, vertigo!

New Symptoms? ______________

____

What I Accomplished Today – Something to Celebrate! ♡

____

____

____

Three Things I am Thankful for Today:

1.
2.
3.

MONTH: January February March April May June July August September October November December

Day: Monday Tuesday Wednesday Thursday Friday Saturday Sunday
Date: ______ **Season:** Summer Autumn/Fall Winter Spring
Temperature: Low ________ High ________
Barometer: 9am__________ 9pm_________ **Humidity** ____________

Sunny	Cloudy	Rain	Showers	Windy
Snow	Storm	Humid	Dry	

Food & Fluid Intake (be mindful of salt):

Breakfast			
Lunch			
Dinner			
Fluid Intake	Water - ________		
Snacks			

Symptoms:

Tinnitus	Vertigo	Drop Attack	Nausea
Anxiety	Brain Fog	Hearing Loss	Hyperacusis
Fatigue	Balance	Co-ordination	Stress
Headache	Migraine	Nystagmus	Disequilibrium
Ear Fullness/ Pressure/Pain	Vision Difficulties	Physical Impairment	Vestibular Migraine
Vomiting	Depression	BPPV*	Diarrhea
PPPD*	Jaw Click/Pain	Neck Pain	Motion Sensitivity
Sweating	Speech Difficulty	Monthly Cycle	

What time did your symptoms start? ______________

Tinnitus: L R How many noises? ________ Loudness Scale: 1 2 3 4 5

Possible Meniere's Symptom Triggers Today:

Physical: ______________

____

____

______________ Pollen, Mold, Dust, Trees, Grass, Ragweed

Visual: ______________

____

____

Emotional: ______________

____

____

What Helped Me?

Medication/s & Time Taken		Other	
		Prayer	Rest
		Meditation	Friend/s
		Self-care	Family
		Exercise	Pet/s
		Mindfulness	Vestibular Rehab
		Gratitude	Hearing Device

Duration of Vertigo ______ minutes ______ hours ______ days

Severity of Vertigo 1 2 3 4 5 - I HATE you, vertigo!

New Symptoms? ______________

____

What I Accomplished Today - Something to Celebrate! ♡

____

____

____

Three Things I am Thankful for Today:

1.
2.
3.

MONTH: January February March April May June July August September October November December

Day: Monday Tuesday Wednesday Thursday Friday Saturday Sunday
Date: ______ **Season:** Summer Autumn/Fall Winter Spring
Temperature: Low ______ High ______
Barometer: 9am______ 9pm______ **Humidity** ______

Sunny	Cloudy	Rain	Showers	Windy
Snow	Storm	Humid	Dry	

Food & Fluid Intake (be mindful of salt):

Breakfast			
Lunch			
Dinner			
Fluid Intake	Water - ______		
Snacks			

Symptoms:

Tinnitus	Vertigo	Drop Attack	Nausea
Anxiety	Brain Fog	Hearing Loss	Hyperacusis
Fatigue	Balance	Co-ordination	Stress
Headache	Migraine	Nystagmus	Disequilibrium
Ear Fullness/ Pressure/Pain	Vision Difficulties	Physical Impairment	Vestibular Migraine
Vomiting	Depression	BPPV*	Diarrhea
PPPD*	Jaw Click/Pain	Neck Pain	Motion Sensitivity
Sweating	Speech Difficulty	Monthly Cycle	

What time did your symptoms start? ____________________

Tinnitus: L R How many noises? ______ Loudness Scale: 1 2 3 4 5

Possible Meniere's Symptom Triggers Today:

Physical: ____________________

____

____

____________________ Pollen, Mold, Dust, Trees, Grass, Ragweed

Visual: ____________________

____

____

Emotional: ____________________

____

____

What Helped Me?

Medication/s & Time Taken		Other	
		Prayer	Rest
		Meditation	Friend/s
		Self-care	Family
		Exercise	Pet/s
		Mindfulness	Vestibular Rehab
		Gratitude	Hearing Device

Duration of Vertigo ______ minutes ______ hours______ days

Severity of Vertigo 1 2 3 4 5 - I HATE you, vertigo!

New Symptoms? ____________________

____

What I Accomplished Today – Something to Celebrate! ♡

____

____

____

Three Things I am Thankful for Today:

1.
2.
3.

MONTH: January February March April May June July August September October November December

Day: Monday Tuesday Wednesday Thursday Friday Saturday Sunday

Date: ______ **Season:** Summer Autumn/Fall Winter Spring

Temperature: Low _______ High _______

Barometer: 9am_______ 9pm_______ **Humidity** ___________

Sunny	Cloudy	Rain	Showers	Windy
Snow	Storm	Humid	Dry	

Food & Fluid Intake (be mindful of salt):

Breakfast			
Lunch			
Dinner			
Fluid Intake	Water - ______		
Snacks			

Symptoms:

Tinnitus	Vertigo	Drop Attack	Nausea
Anxiety	Brain Fog	Hearing Loss	Hyperacusis
Fatigue	Balance	Co-ordination	Stress
Headache	Migraine	Nystagmus	Disequilibrium
Ear Fullness/ Pressure/Pain	Vision Difficulties	Physical Impairment	Vestibular Migraine
Vomiting	Depression	BPPV*	Diarrhea
PPPD*	Jaw Click/Pain	Neck Pain	Motion Sensitivity
Sweating	Speech Difficulty	Monthly Cycle	

What time did your symptoms start? ____________________

Tinnitus: L R How many noises? _______ Loudness Scale: 1 2 3 4 5

Possible Meniere's Symptom Triggers Today:

Physical: ____________________

____

____

____________________ Pollen, Mold, Dust, Trees, Grass, Ragweed

Visual: ____________________

____

____

Emotional: ____________________

____

____

What Helped Me?

Medication/s & Time Taken		Other	
		Prayer	Rest
		Meditation	Friend/s
		Self-care	Family
		Exercise	Pet/s
		Mindfulness	Vestibular Rehab
		Gratitude	Hearing Device

Duration of Vertigo ______ minutes ______ hours______ days

Severity of Vertigo 1 2 3 4 5 - I HATE you, vertigo!

New Symptoms? ____________________

____

What I Accomplished Today - Something to Celebrate! ♡

____

____

____

Three Things I am Thankful for Today:

1.
2.
3.

MONTH: January February March April May June July August September October November December

Day: Monday Tuesday Wednesday Thursday Friday Saturday Sunday
Date: ______ **Season:** Summer Autumn/Fall Winter Spring
Temperature: Low _______ High _______
Barometer: 9am_________ 9pm_________ **Humidity** ___________

Sunny	Cloudy	Rain	Showers	Windy
Snow	Storm	Humid	Dry	

Food & Fluid Intake (be mindful of salt):

Breakfast			
Lunch			
Dinner			
Fluid Intake	Water - ______		
Snacks			

Symptoms:

Tinnitus	Vertigo	Drop Attack	Nausea
Anxiety	Brain Fog	Hearing Loss	Hyperacusis
Fatigue	Balance	Co-ordination	Stress
Headache	Migraine	Nystagmus	Disequilibrium
Ear Fullness/ Pressure/Pain	Vision Difficulties	Physical Impairment	Vestibular Migraine
Vomiting	Depression	BPPV*	Diarrhea
PPPD*	Jaw Click/Pain	Neck Pain	Motion Sensitivity
Sweating	Speech Difficulty	Monthly Cycle	

What time did your symptoms start? ____________________

Tinnitus: L R How many noises? ______ Loudness Scale: 1 2 3 4 5

Possible Meniere's Symptom Triggers Today:

Physical: ____________________

____

____

____________________ Pollen, Mold, Dust, Trees, Grass, Ragweed

Visual: ____________________

____

____

Emotional: ____________________

____

____

What Helped Me?

Medication/s & Time Taken		Other	
		Prayer	Rest
		Meditation	Friend/s
		Self-care	Family
		Exercise	Pet/s
		Mindfulness	Vestibular Rehab
		Gratitude	Hearing Device

Duration of Vertigo ______ minutes ______ hours______ days

Severity of Vertigo 1 2 3 4 5 - I HATE you, vertigo!

New Symptoms? ____________________

____

What I Accomplished Today – Something to Celebrate! ♡

____

____

____

Three Things I am Thankful for Today:

1.
2.
3.

Vertigo. STOP! There will be a cure! Meniere's disease does not define us. Meniere's, I hate you! Tinnitus. MENIERE'S WARRIOR! Hope – there is always hope! Hearing loss. A cure will be found! Imbalance. Take each day one at a time. BREATHE. Create moments. Find things to be thankful for. Ear pain. You will overcome. Good things are coming. Research. Meniere's, your time is UP! Vertigo. There will be a cure! Meniere's disease does not define us. Meniere's, I hate you! Tinnitus. MENIERE'S WARRIOR! Hope – there is always hope! Hearing loss. A cure will be found! Imbalance. Take each day one at a time. BREATHE. Create moments. Find things to be thankful for. Ear pain. You will overcome. Good things are coming. Research. Meniere's, your time is UP! Vertigo. There will be a cure! Meniere's disease does not define us. Meniere's, I hate you! Tinnitus. MENIERE'S WARRIOR! Hope – there is always hope! Hearing loss. A cure will be found! Imbalance. Take each day one at a time. BREATHE. Create moments. Find things to be thankful for. Ear pain. You will overcome. Good things are coming. Research. Meniere's, your time is UP! Vertigo. There will be a cure! Meniere's disease does not define us. Meniere's, I hate you! Tinnitus. MENIERE'S WARRIOR! Hope, there is always hope! We will be cured! BREATHE...vertigo. STOP! There will be a cure! Meniere's disease does not define us. Meniere's, I hate you! Tinnitus. MENIERE'S WARRIOR! Hope – there is always hope! Hearing loss. A cure will be found! Imbalance. Take each day one at a time. BREATHE. Create moments. Find things to be thankful for. Ear pain. You will overcome. Good things are coming. Research. Meniere's, your time is UP! Vertigo. There will be a cure! Meniere's disease does not define us. Meniere's, I hate you! Tinnitus. MENIERE'S WARRIOR! Hope – there is always hope! Hearing loss. A cure will be found! Imbalance. Take each day one at a time. BREATHE. Create moments. Find things to be thankful for. Ear pain. You will overcome. Good things are coming. Research. Meniere's, your time is UP! Vertigo. There will be a cure! Meniere's disease does not define us. Meniere's, I hate you! Tinnitus. MENIERE'S WARRIOR! Hope – there is always hope! Hearing loss. A cure will be found! Imbalance. Take each day one at a time. BREATHE. Create moments. Find things to be thankful for. Ear pain. You will overcome. Good things are coming. Research. Meniere's, your time is UP! Vertigo. There will be a cure! Meniere's disease does not define us. Meniere's, I hate you! Tinnitus. MENIERE'S WARRIOR! Hope, there is always hope! We will be cured! BREATHE...vertigo. STOP! There will be a cure! Meniere's disease does not define us. Meniere's, I hate you! Tinnitus. MENIERE'S WARRIOR! Hope – there is always hope! Hearing loss. A cure will be found! Imbalance. Take each day one at a time. BREATHE. Create moments. Find things to be thankful for. Ear pain. You will overcome. Good things are coming. Research. Meniere's, your time is UP! Vertigo. **There will be a cure!**

Vertigo. STOP! There will be a cure! Meniere's disease does not define us. Meniere's, I hate you! Tinnitus. MENIERE'S WARRIOR! Hope – there is always hope! Hearing loss. A cure will be found! Imbalance. Take each day one at a time. BREATHE. Create moments. Find things to be thankful for. Ear pain. You will overcome. Good things are coming. Research. Meniere's, your time is UP! Vertigo. There will be a cure! Meniere's disease does not define us. Meniere's, I hate you! Tinnitus. MENIERE'S WARRIOR! Hope – there is always hope! Hearing loss. A cure will be found! Imbalance. Take each day one at a time. BREATHE. Create moments. Find things to be thankful for. Ear pain. You will overcome. Good things are coming. Research. Meniere's, your time is UP! Vertigo. There will be a cure! Meniere's disease does not define us. Meniere's, I hate you! Tinnitus. MENIERE'S WARRIOR! Hope – there is always hope! Hearing loss. A cure will be found! Imbalance. Take each day one at a time. BREATHE. Create moments. Find things to be thankful for. Ear pain. You will overcome. Good things are coming. Research. Meniere's, your time is UP! Vertigo. There will be a cure! Meniere's disease does not define us. Meniere's, I hate you! Tinnitus. MENIERE'S WARRIOR! Hope, there is always hope! We will be cured! BREATHE...vertigo. STOP! There will be a cure! Meniere's disease does not define us. Meniere's, I hate you! Tinnitus. MENIERE'S WARRIOR! Hope – there is always hope! Hearing loss. A cure will be found! Imbalance. Take each day one at a time. BREATHE. Create moments. Find things to be thankful for. Ear pain. You will overcome. Good things are coming. Research. Meniere's, your time is UP! Vertigo. There will be a cure! Meniere's disease does not define us. Meniere's, I hate you! Tinnitus. MENIERE'S WARRIOR! Hope – there is always hope! Hearing loss. A cure will be found! Imbalance. Take each day one at a time. BREATHE. Create moments. Find things to be thankful for. Ear pain. You will overcome. Good things are coming. Research. Meniere's, your time is UP! Vertigo. There will be a cure! Meniere's disease does not define us. Meniere's, I hate you! Tinnitus. MENIERE'S WARRIOR! Hope – there is always hope! Hearing loss. A cure will be found! Imbalance. Take each day one at a time. BREATHE. Create moments. Find things to be thankful for. Ear pain. You will overcome. Good things are coming. Research. Meniere's, your time is UP! Vertigo. There will be a cure! Meniere's disease does not define us. Meniere's, I hate you! Tinnitus. MENIERE'S WARRIOR! Hope, there is always hope! We will be cured! BREATHE...vertigo. STOP! There will be a cure! Meniere's disease does not define us. Meniere's, I hate you! Tinnitus. MENIERE'S WARRIOR! Hope – there is always hope! Hearing loss. A cure will be found! Imbalance. Take each day one at a time. BREATHE. Create moments. Find things to be thankful for. Ear pain. You will overcome. Good things are coming. Research. Meniere's, your time is UP! Vertigo. **There will be a cure!**

My Action Plan to Conquer Meniere's Disease

What I Have Learned About Myself

I'm Thankful for ...

www.ingramcontent.com/pod-product-compliance
Lightning Source LLC
LaVergne TN
LVHW041910270126
830598LV00023B/2555

* 9 7 8 0 6 4 5 1 5 8 1 0 6 *